Improving Nursing Home Care of the Dying

DATE DUE

D1360176

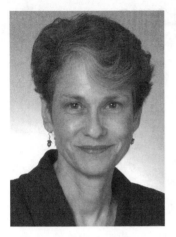

Martha L. Henderson, MSN, DrMin, is a geriatric nurse practitioner (GNP) on the faculty of the University of North Carolina School of Medicine, Program on Aging, and School of Nursing. She was named a Project on Death in America faculty scholar by the Soros Foundation's Open Society Institute. In addition to her ongoing work on improving end-of-life care in nursing homes, she is currently researching a model of employing geriatric nurse practitioners as end-of-life care facilitators for community-dwelling individuals with advanced chronic illness. She serves on the UNC Hospitals Ethics Committee and consultation team and helps educate health care providers in how to deal with ethical dilemmas at the end of life.

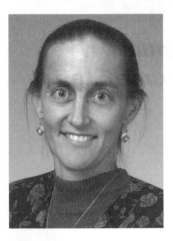

Laura Hanson, MD, MPH, is an Associate Professor in the Department of Medicine at the School of Medicine, University of North Carolina Chapel Hill and practices Geriatric Medicine at the University of North Carolina School of Medicine. She directs the interdisciplinary Geriatric Evaluation Clinic and co-directs the Pain and Symptom Care Program, a clinical palliative care service for UNC Hospitals. Dr. Hanson graduated from Harvard Medical School and was awarded an MPH degree in Epidemiology from the UNC School of Public Health. She is a member of the Core Faculty for the Robert Wood Johnson Clinical Scholars Program at UNC and serves on Ethics Committees for UNC Hospitals, the Society of General Internal Medicine, and the American Geriatrics Society.

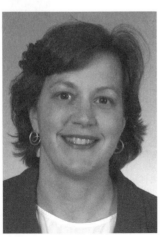

Kimberly Reynolds, MPA, serves as director of the Project to Improve End-of-Life Care in Nursing Homes and is principal investigator of a study exploring racial disparities in end-of-life care. She is a recent recipient of the Gordon DeFriese Career Development in Aging Award from North Carolina's Institute on Aging; she holds a National Research Service Award Traineeship from the Agency for Health Care Policy and Research and serves as a pre-doctoral fellow at the Cecil G. Sheps Center for Health Services Research, University of North Carolina at Chapel Hill. Ms. Reynolds has worked as a health policy analyst at the United States Senate. She is finishing a PhD in health behavior and health education at the University of North Carolina's School of Public Health.

Improving Nursing Home Care of the Dying

A Training Manual For Nursing Home Staff

Martha L. Henderson, MSN, Dr Min
Laura C. Hanson, MPH, MD
Kimberly S. Reynolds, MPA

 Springer Publishing Company

Springer Publishing Company, Inc.
536 Broadway
New York, NY 10012-3955

Acquisitions Editor: Helvi Gold
Production Editor: Janice Stangel
Cover design by Joanne E. Honigman

04 05/5 4 3

Library of Congress Cataloging-in-Publication Data

Henderson, Martha L., MSN.
    Improving nursing home care of the dying : a training manual for nursing home staff / Martha L. Henderson, Laura C. Hanson, Kimberly S. Reynolds.
        p. cm.
    Includes bibliographical references and index.
    ISBN 0-8261-1925-5
    1. Nursing home patients—Care Handbooks, manuals, etc.
    2. Terminal care—Handbooks, manuals, etc. 3. Aged—Nursing home care—Handbooks, manuals, etc. I. Hanson, Laura C. II. Reynolds, Kimberly S. III. Title.

RC954.3 .H466 2003
362.1'75—dc21   2002036657

Printed in the United States of America by Vicks Lithograph & Printing Corporation.

Contents

Foreword

Embracing Nursing Homes as the Place of Care and Site of Death for Frail, Older Americans

Increasingly, nursing homes are the place of care and where older, frail persons die in the United States of America. In 1997, one in four persons with chronic illnesses died in a nursing home, with some states having more than one in three persons dying in a nursing home. Now is the time to embrace the nursing home as an important place of care and site of death for older Americans. This trend will only increase with growing numbers of elderly persons and current financial incentives for hospitals to discharge persons "quicker and sicker." Urgently, we must insure that staff in long term care facilities have the needed knowledge, skills, and tools to provide competent, coordinated, and compassionate end of life care. *Improving Nursing Home Care of the Dying: A Training Manual for Nursing Home Staff* is an important resource to provide nursing homes, hospices, and palliative care teams with the training material to educate staff how to provide care to frail, older persons living in nursing homes.

In eight didactic sessions, Martha Henderson, Laura Hanson, and Kimberly Reynolds provide sage advice, assessment tools, and practical exercises to educate staff about care of the dying. The challenges to providing high quality end of life care in nursing homes are substantial. Unlike persons dying of cancer, professionals caring for frail, older dying persons are faced with blurred boundaries and, often, multiple "close calls" where, for example, the person with advanced dementia could have died with this episode of pneumonia. There are no easy answers. As families go through the difficult process of hope and eventual realization that one's relative will never again be the father, mother, or other close person that they knew growing up, they need consistent and clear communication from caregivers who understand this complicated path—one that is painful, confusing, and too often, one that families face alone and without adequate counsel. The enclosed case histories help staff to understand and aid families going through this difficult process. Practical communication tips help all staff, including nursing assistants, support the families of dying nursing home residents as well as raise important decisions that nursing home staff and families must make. The multidisciplinary focus in this training manual outlines important roles for all health care providers, including the certified nursing assistant. CNAs provide the bulk of care and caring for older nursing home residents. Often, these persons are never thanked nor their professionalism acknowledged.

Nursing homes are the final safety net for frail, older persons. Often, they are faced with conflicting regulatory goals—preserving function yet respecting resident autonomy for a peaceful death. These institutions take on this challenge in a time of declining reimbursement, increased regulation, and low esteem from other sectors of the health care industry. Now is the time to embrace nursing homes—efforts such as those of the authors and others are key to ensure that our oldest generation receives the competent and compassionate care that they deserve.

Joan M Teno, M.D., M.S.
December 30, 2002

Preface

One in five people in the United States will die in a nursing home. This manual is dedicated to improving the care of those individuals. Nursing homes have the potential to provide excellent end-of-life care. Many residents live in nursing homes for months or even years, permitting staff to know them well. These types of long-term relationships are unique among health care settings, and they are a great asset in providing highly individualized and effective care. Residents of nursing homes can find physical and emotional comfort, support for their families, and respect for their wishes as they face the final phase of life. Nursing home staff often take pride in the care they give to residents who are dying, and the staff provide nearly all terminal care for residents, assisted by hospice or other palliative care services in a small minority of cases. Education of nursing home staff is therefore an essential aspect of any program of clinical care for the dying.

Residents of nursing homes usually die of advanced chronic illnesses, such as heart failure, chronic lung disease, and neurological diseases such as stroke or Alzheimer's dementia. The course of these illnesses is less predictable than the final stages of terminal cancer. Physicians and nurses face great uncertainty about the timing of death for this population, although they may recognize that some residents are declining or failing to respond to treatment. This uncertainty means that planning for the end of life should begin early for this population. To ensure good care at the end of life, all nursing home residents need attention to their physical, emotional, and spiritual needs, as well as an opportunity to voice preferences about life-sustaining treatments. For some residents, palliation of symptoms and assurance of comfort will become the focus of a good plan of care.

What constitutes high-quality care for residents dying in long-term care facilities? Researchers have asked individuals with life-limiting illnesses and found that they want excellent symptom control, avoidance of a prolonged dying process, a feeling of control, attention to loved ones, and an emphasis on the quality of daily living while dying. Experts in nursing home care emphasize quality standards for pain and symptom relief, support to meet personal care needs, effective communication of treatment preferences, services to meet emotional and spiritual needs of residents and families, and an organizational culture that rewards teamwork and facilitates communication about end-of-life care.

Education can be more effective when it builds on staff members' wealth of clinical experience to improve specific knowledge and skills. We developed this curriculum while working with experienced staff from nine nursing homes, collaborating in a multiyear project to evaluate the care needs of dying nursing home residents and the educational needs of staff. The resulting book covers eight topics in end-of-life and palliative care in a long-term care setting. These topics are essential, but not exclusive, content for nursing home staff caring for residents facing the final phase of life. The book may be used as a curriculum taught over time in a nursing home. Alternatively, each chapter may be used alone to fit a particular need of residents and staff. The educational materials are designed to engage the learner and help nursing home staff apply what they have learned. Each chapter contains core content and homework assignments that requires learners to put their new knowledge into practice. Most chapters also provide clinical cases to prompt group discussion.

This educational program is designed for interdisciplinary teaching that will model and foster teamwork in caring for residents at the end of their lives. Each individual and each discipline within a long-term care facility provides a valuable and unique perspective on how to contribute to excellent care of residents. The team needs to hear each other to grow in appreciation and to strengthen cooperation in their work together.

Administrative support of this educational endeavor is essential to its success. The nursing home administrator, the medical director, and the director of nursing are important authorities in promoting improved care of dying residents and offering staff the opportunity to grow in this area. Paying for staff to come in early or stay late to attend sessions, or scheduling extra workers on the day of the sessions, provides tangible evidence of support. If a nursing home administrator attends the training sessions and offers a statement of support and commitment to the facility's educational effort, it will bolster staff participation. We also encourage facilities to reward every staff person who attends all the sessions or who participates actively in the training program. This recognition will increase pride and provide mentorship for others who want to increase their knowledge and skills in end-of-life care.

The most helpful facilitators or teachers of this material are individuals who have experience working with dying long-term care residents and who also have skills and experience in teaching. Ideally, hospice nurses and social workers located near the nursing home may be willing to teach this curriculum either on a contractual or a volunteer basis. Advantages of this arrangement are that not only are hospice personnel experts in end-of-life care, but such an educational endeavor between nursing homes and hospices builds relationships, trust, and the opportunity for hospice referrals and consultation when appropriate. Other facilitators for this curriculum may include staff development coordinators within nursing homes. They may lead the sessions, use nursing home leaders within their own facilities, or solicit help from local professional resources such as university or community college nursing faculty, hospital chaplains and social workers, or religious leaders from the community.

A critical component for successful training is an individual who will take responsibility for scheduling, arranging, and publicizing the sessions. Frequent communication with staff about these sessions is essential. Posting the dates and titles of the sessions well ahead of time and then distributing flyers the week before will help build interest and facilitate attendance. Reminders to all staff the day before and the day of the sessions will increase participation. Ideally, sessions can be taught for each shift, but an alternative is videotaping the daytime sessions and then allowing evening and night shift workers to view the videos at a quiet time. Printed copies of the curriculum should be available to every learner.

We hope this book will serve as a resource not only for improving staff competence in end-of-life care, but also for instilling confidence and commitment to the goal of a good death for every resident.

Martha Henderson
Laura C. Hanson
Kimberly S. Reynolds
June 15, 2002

Acknowledgments

We initially began this work with generous support from the Soros Foundation/Open Society Institute's *Project on Death in America*. Funding from this dynamic organization allowed us to develop and test an innovative educational program to improve care of the dying in nursing homes. The Duke University Institute for Care at the End of Life provided additional funding to disseminate the resulting educational materials in book form so that others working in long-term care settings could benefit. Funding from the Duke Endowment has enabled us to continue to implement and further refine our curriculum. We are also grateful to the Robert Wood Johnson Foundation's *Community-State Partnerships to Improve End-of-Life Care* and the Carolinas Center for Hospice and End of Life Care for their support and guidance.

Notes for the Facilitator

Nursing home staff are being asked to care for more and more residents who are dying. Most people want a peaceful, comfortable death, and helping them to achieve this is a challenge and privilege for staff. These educational sessions are designed to help nursing home staff meet this challenge and give competent and compassionate care.

These materials ideally will be used as a comprehensive training course but may be used for individual sessions. Each module includes a presentation, a case for discussion, handouts that summarize the content, and a homework assignment so learners can take practical actions based on what they have learned. You should plan 45 to 90 minutes of teaching and discussion to cover each session. Longer sessions may be divided in half by using the presentation and homework assignment initially, followed by a second session for case discussion and discussion of learners' experiences with the homework. Sessions may include all types of staff, although the pain management and the emotional and spiritual care modules have some separate materials for aides and licensed personnel. The module on recognizing the final phase of life is also divided, with material on caring for dying individuals (primarily for nurses and nursing assistants) and material on prognosis (for physicians, physician assistants, and nurse practitioners).

The following are general issues to keep in mind when presenting these sessions:

1. As facilitator you should read through the module before each session and plan a presentation appropriate to your learners. Check the module's bibliography for materials you may wish to read or share.
2. Talking about death can generate feelings that may be intense. Remind the group in each session that it is normal to feel sad when talking about death. You or the facility social worker should be available to talk with participants after the session if needed.

3. Each facility has its own approach to the subject of dying and residents' deaths. Be aware of the general attitude and approach to death and dying in the facility where you are teaching. Ask about this and find out how staff feel about the facility's approach. Be alert to opportunities to help foster an open and supportive environment.

4. Some people have cultural or religious beliefs about how to care for someone who is dying. It is your job to explain that differences exist and encourage an attitude of tolerance and learning from each other.

5. Educational sessions can be used to create new connections with community resources. For example, you can invite hospice nurses to coteach the session on pain management, or ask a hospice chaplain or local clergy to talk about the spiritual needs of dying residents.

6. Adults learn best from their own experiences. Plan time in the session for questions and discussion, and practice your presentation ahead of time.

7. Prior to each session, photocopy the corresponding handouts from *Appendix E* so that you can give copies to each participant. (Copy at 121% enlargement for a full-size reproduction.) Distributing summaries of each session's highlights will aid in retention of the material and will allow participants to share their knowledge with other staff members. Assign the homework to encourage participants to practice what they have just learned. Be available to talk with them about their experiences.

8. Make it easy and fun to come to sessions—provide refreshments, educational credit, and make sure that people are given work coverage during the time they are in sessions.

Envisioning a Good Death

OVERVIEW

Welcome to this first session on improving nursing home care of the dying. This session is for us to dream—to create a vision of what an ideal death would be like in our facility. We'll spend time imagining how we can create a comforting and caring place for people to die.

> **Instructions to Facilitator:** Dim the lights, create a comfortable environment. Play soft instrumental music if desired. Read the following statements and questions slowly, pausing between each part to allow participants to reflect. This presentation should take 10–15 minutes, allowing extensive time for discussion. *Time estimate: 45 minutes.*

❐ Close your eyes. Relax. Take slow deep breaths.

❐ Connect with your heart. Recall memories of a good death that you have witnessed and what made it so. Or think about your dream of a good death for yourself or a loved one.

❐ Recall memories of a death that affected you strongly. Choose one person or one story to focus on. This could be someone from your past—a resident you've cared for, a family member, or a friend. Or create a vision of a good death you see in the future for someone you love.

❐ Imagine that person is dying in a room in your nursing home. If the person had a good death, think about what made it so. If not, think about how you wish it could have been.

❐ See the dying person's face. Who is this person to you? What is the expression on their face?

❐ See where the person is in their room in the nursing home. What are their immediate surroundings like? What are the favorite things they want to have with them to comfort them?

❐ What is the person listening to? What are their favorite sounds, music, and voices?

❐ Who else is there? Who do they want with them during this time? How do you interact with them?

❐ What does the person need now, as they are dying? What do they ask for? What do they need that they can't or won't ask for? How do you know what they need?

Instructions to Facilitator: Ask the participants to come back together as they take some deep breaths. Tell them you will turn the lights back on. Begin a discussion of people's visions. Ask participants to share their thoughts briefly, so that several people will have time to talk.

QUESTIONS FOR DISCUSSION

❐ Would someone share their vision of a good death with the group?

❐ What factors contributed to good deaths?

❐ How can we meet all aspects of the resident's dying experience, including:

- physical needs: helping the resident be physically comfortable

- emotional needs: listening for feelings

- social needs: encouraging relationships with others

- spiritual needs: supporting resident's beliefs and practices

Instructions to Facilitator: Finish the session by reading aloud or asking a volunteer from the group to read aloud the conclusion presented below. Then hand out and explain the homework.

CONCLUSION

As caregivers, we have a special privilege and responsibility to help residents finish their final journey well. When we visualize what a good death might look like, we will be better able to help residents achieve a good dying experience.

ANNOTATED BIBLIOGRAPHY

Note to Facilitator: Before you present this session, if you would like to learn more about envisioning a good death, we suggest the following articles.

Hanson, L. C., Henderson, M., & Menon, M. (2002). As individual as death itself: A focus group study of terminal care in nursing homes. *Journal of Palliative Medicine, 5,* 117–125.
   The authors conducted focus groups with nursing home staff and physicians, asking the participants to define a good death in a long-term-care setting and to describe the factors that promote or hinder good care for dying nursing home residents. Nursing home staff encouraged highly individualized care, including continuity of relationships between residents and staff members; teamwork among staff, physicians, and family members; and comprehensive advance care planning as methods of providing high-quality end-of-life care. Nursing home staff documented that their experience in providing care and their personal relationships with residents contributed to improved end-of-life care in their facilities.
Lethem, W. (November 3, 1999). Nursing home nurses deliver palliative care. *Nursing Times, 95,* 54–55.
   This short, easy-to-read article in a British nursing journal discusses five aspects of palliative care in nursing homes: focusing on quality of life and good symptom control, caring for the whole person, including friends and family, respecting resident autonomy and choice, and emphasizing open communication and teamwork among family and nursing home staff. The author gives suggestions for how to achieve each of these goals.
Reynolds, K. S., Henderson, M., Schulman, A., & Hanson, L. C. (2002). Needs of the dying in nursing homes. *Journal of Palliative Medicine, 5,* 895–901.

The authors of this article interviewed nursing home staff and family members of recently deceased nursing home residents, asking them about the physical and emotional symptoms, unmet treatment needs, and quality of the dying experience for the deceased residents. They concluded that dying residents need attention not only to traditional palliative care services such as pain and symptom control, but that in a nursing home setting, residents near the end of life have a particular need for emotional and spiritual support and for help with personal cleanliness.

Steinhauser, K. E., Clipp, E. C., McNeilly, M., Christakis, N. A., McInyre, L. M., & Tulsky, J. A. (2000). In search of a good death: Observations of patients, families, and providers. *Annals of Internal Medicine, 132,* 825–832.

This research team conducted focus groups with individuals near the end of life, recently bereaved family members, and people who work with the dying, to gather descriptions of the components of a good death. Six major themes emerged from the group discussions: (1) pain and symptom management; (2) clear decision making (for example, advance directives); (3) preparation for death; (4) completion, including a focus on spiritual issues, life review, and the opportunity to resolve conflicts and say good-bye; (5) contributing to others; and (6) affirmation of the whole person, with health care providers focusing not just on the 'disease' but on personal relationships.

Your turn. (July, 1998). *Journal of Gerontological Nursing, 24,* 47–52.

This journal's editors asked the readers to respond to the question, "In your practice, what experiences of patients and family members could be classified as a good death or a positive process of dying?" The editors received numerous eloquent responses from nurses who care for dying nursing home residents. Descriptions of "good deaths" included statements such as: "We have several CNAs who feel comfortable reading or reciting scripture, singing gospel hymns, and/or sitting with residents who are at death's door. Residents leave this world in peace with their 'extended family' at their bedside." "The [nurses] massaged the patient's back and held his hand until the family arrived. [They] were able to comfort the family members by listening to them, by explaining the imminent death of their father, and by crying together."

2

Recognizing the Final Phase of Life

OVERVIEW

This session focuses on identifying when a resident is nearing death. We have to recognize the possibility that someone is dying before we can give him or her special care. We will discuss ways to predict death and recognize the signs of active dying. The session will also cover some of the physical and emotional symptoms that residents may exhibit as they prepare for their deaths. The goal of this session is for us to be able to determine better when residents are nearing the final stages of life so that we can provide high-quality end-of-life care, focusing on promoting comfort and quality of life.

> **Instructions to Facilitator:** Discuss the following topics with session participants, taking questions and comments as they arise. Note that this module includes some materials relevant primarily to MDs, NPs, PAs, and licensed nursing staff. *Time estimate: 60 minutes.*

IDENTIFYING RESIDENTS WHO ARE NEARING DEATH

We can create special care plans for residents in the final phase of life. Residents who are candidates for a discussion of the option of palliative care (comfort care) include:

❏   Any resident with a life expectancy of less than six months.

❏   Any resident about whom you can say, "If she died within the next year, I would not be surprised."

❐ Any resident with an incurable, progressive disease (for example, advanced Alzheimer's or congestive heart failure with severe symptoms).

❐ Any resident who elects a palliative or comfort care approach.

See *Appendix B* for examples of comfort care planning forms and possible comfort care orders.

HOW DO WE DETERMINE THAT SOMEONE IS DYING?

❐ *Identifying Terminal Illness:* A doctor or nurse can often predict that death will occur *within months* from the resident's current illness, if the illness follows its usual course. This kind of illness is called a terminal illness, and can be thought of as the beginning of the final phase of a person's life. Communication of this awareness of approaching death is the critical first step to permit residents and their families to prepare for death and receive appropriate care.

❐ *Preparing:* As a resident experiences significant and progressive decline, he may recognize he is dying and begin to prepare for it. This personal preparation *can happen at any time, or never happen.* A person who is preparing for death may feel many strong emotions, especially if he receives a terminal diagnosis—denial, anger, bargaining, depression, and acceptance are emotional stages experienced by some, but not all, dying persons. CNAs and nurses are often the first to hear about or see evidence of this preparation.

❐ *Active Dying:* Caregivers can recognize physical signs that indicate death will occur *within hours or days.* These physical signs may occur after diagnosis of a terminal illness or in the absence of such a diagnosis. While actively dying residents have special care needs, they may be unable to communicate at this stage of their illness.

Information for Licensed Nursing Staff, MDs, NPs, and PAs

Note to Facilitator: The following section (on identifying prognosis) is useful primarily to nurse practitioners, physician assistants, physicians, and licensed nursing staff. Adjust the amount of time you spend on this topic depending on your particular audience.

HOW DO WE RECOGNIZE RESIDENTS WHO ARE TERMINALLY ILL OR IN THE FINAL PHASE OF LIFE?

☐ We can never identify all residents who are dying, but some clinical guidelines can help.

☐ The Flacker mortality score (see *Appendix A*) uses Minimum Data Set (MDS) information to estimate the likelihood of dying within 1 year based on:

- functional dependency

- weight loss of 10 pounds in 6 months or 5 pounds in 1 month

- presence of congestive heart failure

- shortness of breath

- swallowing problems

- male gender

- advanced age

- low body mass index

☐ Morrison and colleagues (see annotated bibliography) studied patients with severe dementia (similar to hospice guidelines) who were hospitalized for pneumonia or hip fracture, and found a 50% mortality rate at 6 months.

☐ Guidelines developed by the National Hospice and Palliative Care Organization (NHPCO) provide disease-specific criteria for a probable death within 6 months. To obtain this useful work, contact NHPCO and ask for their publication *Guidelines for Determining Prognosis in Selected Non-Cancer Diseases.* [See *Appendix*

8

Improving Nursing Home Care of the Dying

A for a one-page summary of these guidelines.] Information on local hospice services is also available from the NHPCO. Contact:

The National Hospice and Palliative Care Organization
1700 Diagonal Road, Suite 300
Alexandria, VA 22314
1-800-658-8898
www.NHPCO.org

❒ Refer residents for hospice evaluation when you suspect they are likely to die within 6 months; the hospice team can help to clarify predicted life expectancy as part of their evaluation.

❒ Be humble. Predicting when death will occur is often difficult, and you should communicate this to residents and their families.

HOW DO WE COMMUNICATE PROGNOSIS AND BEGIN A DISCUSSION OF PALLIATIVE CARE GOALS?

Many patients and their families prefer palliative care with an emphasis on comfort and quality of life once they know that death is near. Effective communication of prognosis is the critical first step toward good care at the end of life.

❒ Begin by asking for their concerns and fears—what do they think is happening to the resident as the illness progresses?

❒ Provide them with the best estimate of prognosis you can.

■ Because the exact timing of death for any individual is difficult to predict, it is inaccurate to predict death within a very narrowly defined time period. It is more helpful (and more accurate) to say "From what I know about the course of inoperable heart disease with severe heart failure, he is likely to have only months left to live—it would be unusual for someone as ill as he is to be alive a year from now."

❒ Provide them with information on what to expect—how will the illness unfold over the coming months?

■ "Patients with end-stage Alzheimer's disease usually have several infections like pneumonia or urinary tract infections prior to death. Often one of these infections will be the final cause of death. These patients also typically have some difficulty swallowing, and they appear to lose interest in taking food or water by mouth. At the very end, they are often quite peaceful and calm."

❐   Let the resident and the family know that you sympathize with their fear or grief—"I know that this is hard to hear, and I am sorry that modern medicine cannot cure or stop the progression of this difficult illness."

❐   As you discuss treatments and care with the resident and family, encourage them to discuss what is most important to them now. Encourage them to do advance care planning, including making treatment decisions, so that all are prepared when the time of dying comes.

❐   Offer them hope in the form of effective palliative treatments, and comfort in your continued interest and willingness to provide care during the dying process. Let them ask questions or express fears.

  ■   "When someone is facing the final months of life, they often fear that they will suffer severe pain or be neglected. I will come to see you at the nursing home any time you need extra help with symptoms of this illness. I know many treatments that can make you more comfortable during this difficult time."

  ■   "Are there any special concerns or fears you have about facing death? Are there any questions you want to ask me?"

Information for All Nursing Home Staff

> **Note to Facilitator:** The following sections (on the value of hospice, resident behaviors shortly before death, comfort measures, and conclusions) are appropriate for all nursing home staff.

HOW CAN HOSPICE CARE BENEFIT NURSING HOME RESIDENTS, THEIR FAMILIES, AND THE STAFF WHO CARE FOR THEM?

❐   Hospice care is specialized care provided by an interdisciplinary team to residents who meet medical criteria for terminal illness.

The hospice care team will work with you to provide expert pain and symptom management, emotional and spiritual care, and supportive care after death for the resident's family and for nursing home staff who are grieving.

❏ Studies of nursing home residents receiving hospice care show:

■ improved family satisfaction with end-of-life care

■ improved control of pain

■ decreased use of hospital transfers, tube feeding, and physical restraints

❏ Some local hospice organizations offer palliative care consultation services for residents who are not eligible for or do not want to enroll in hospice.

❏ In addition to direct care of residents, the hospice team can also provide consultation, support, and education for nursing home staff who provide palliative care.

WHAT BEHAVIORS MIGHT NURSING HOME RESIDENTS EXHIBIT IN THE WEEKS TO MONTHS BEFORE DEATH?

❏ Social withdrawal, personal reflection, less communication or a desire to address old conflicts.

❏ Increased sleep and decreased intake of food and water.

❏ Postponing death until meaningful events occur (for example, birth of a great-grandchild, visit from a family member).

❏ Saying good-bye, looking for permission to die, expressions of soul weariness—"I'm tired of living"—although it is important to consider new physical symptoms or depression as possible causes of these changes.

IDENTIFYING AND COMFORTING RESIDENTS WHO ARE ACTIVELY DYING

What are the signs of active dying, in the days and hours before death? How can nursing home staff create comfort during active dying?

We can all help families by recognizing, acknowledging, and explaining these changes when death is near.

❏ *Coolness*—extremities cool to touch, dusky, mottled, purplish color on extremities with pale or gray-blue nailbeds

  ▪ provide warm blankets or clothing

❏ *Less alert*—drowsy, sleepy, hard to awaken, eyes open but not focused

  ▪ always assume the resident can hear, smell, and feel

  ▪ talk and touch gently, respectfully

  ▪ don't talk in the room as if the resident is absent

❏ *"Terminal alertness"*—a spurt of energy and mental clarity shortly before dying

  ▪ educate family about this possibility

  ▪ encourage family to take this time for close communication and good-byes

❏ *Disorientation and delirium*—waxing and waning confusion, hallucinations

  ▪ reassure; offer orienting information if that is calming, or go along with the resident's reality if that is more helpful

  ▪ educate the family that there may be a period of "terminal alertness"

  ▪ take advantage of all opportunities to communicate and love

  ▪ if very distressed, consider antipsychotic medication

❏ *Restlessness*—picking, pulling, turning

  ▪ use gentle massage, reassuring talk, or music

  ▪ distinguish from delirium, pain, or inadequate oxygen

❏ *Decreased intake*—diminished appetite, thirst, and ability to take food

  ▪ offer refreshing tastes, sips, ice chips, mouth care

  ▪ if unable to swallow, give mouth care only

  ▪ note that this is natural and usually does not cause suffering

❐ *Incontinence and decreased urine output*

- use incontinence pads; consider a Foley or condom catheter for comfort

❐ *Distressing physical appearance or odor*

- increase intensity of personal care for cleanliness

- provide hair and facial care to create a more familiar appearance

- use oil of wintergreen in room for odor control

- bandage or cover distorted areas of the body

❐ *Vital signs*—decreased blood pressure, variable pulse, respirations, and temperature

- stop measuring, unless the information is needed to inform family about approaching death; this may allow aides time to provide other comfort care

❐ *Breathing pattern*—labored, irregular, cyclical, or shallow breathing may occur

- give oxygen, low-dose morphine

- elevate head

- give hyoscyamine or atropine for thick secretions

- give morphine or nebulized albuterol for wheezing

- explain and reassure family

CONCLUSIONS

❐ Predicting death is difficult, but nursing home staff and physicians should work together to try to estimate and communicate a resident's prognosis.

❐ Estimating and communicating prognosis will improve care planning and help to prepare residents and family members.

❐ Hospice or palliative care referral can help clarify a terminal prognosis and create effective care plans to provide good end-of-life care.

❐ Nursing home staff can recognize active dying in the last days or hours of life and initiate effective symptom management for comfort and supportive care.

Instructions to Facilitator: After going through the material above, move on to the case-based example. Have someone in the group read the example and issues aloud, pausing for discussion along the way. Conclude the session by reading through and discussing the action plan and handing out the homework.

An Example for Group Discussion

Case-Based Example: Mr. Jones

Mr. Jones was admitted to the nursing home three months ago with lung cancer and emphysema in addition to mild dementia. He received rehabilitative care in the nursing home but was discharged with home hospice based on his diagnosis and failure to improve.

The patient's son is his surrogate decisionmaker and cared for him while at home. He quickly found his father's care needs overwhelming, and after two days the patient was rehospitalized with respiratory distress and dehydration. When discharged again to the nursing home, the son expected another attempt at rehabilitation. However, after a month's time the resident was weaker, had lost weight, and his baseline mild disorientation had worsened. The son became angry about his father's failure to improve and asked the staff to consider additional IV hydration and hospitalization.

Staff believe that Mr. Jones has had an adequate trial of rehabilitation and now think he is actively dying. They also think Mr. Jones understands this fact, although he hasn't said so. The son is hesitant to agree to a DNR order, and the physician, who has never met the son, does not want to become involved with an angry family member. Nursing home staff have asked the hospice team to do an evaluation, but the local hospice is uncomfortable about getting involved if the son refuses their services.

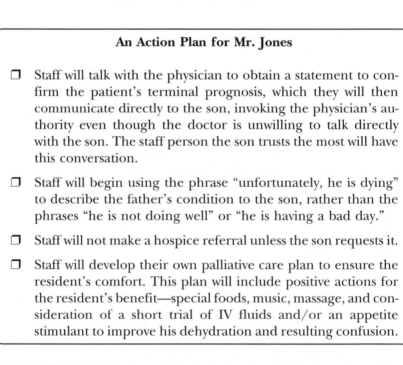

Issues to Consider

❐ *The younger Mr. Jones does not agree that his father has a termi-nal illness.*

❐ *Communication is needed to clarify that the failure of the rehabilitation is not due to staff incompetence but rather to the severity of the resident's progressive and terminal illness.*

❐ *Nursing home staff wish to have a DNR order, and they are afraid IV fluids would worsen Mr. Jones's respiratory distress.*

❐ *The hospice and the physician are not providing support or assistance to staff.*

Stop: Discuss the above case before continuing. How would you propose treating Mr. Jones and working with his son to resolve these issues?

An Action Plan for Mr. Jones

❐ Staff will talk with the physician to obtain a statement to con-firm the patient's terminal prognosis, which they will then communicate directly to the son, invoking the physician's au-thority even though the doctor is unwilling to talk directly with the son. The staff person the son trusts the most will have this conversation.

❐ Staff will begin using the phrase "unfortunately, he is dying" to describe the father's condition to the son, rather than the phrases "he is not doing well" or "he is having a bad day."

❐ Staff will not make a hospice referral unless the son requests it.

❐ Staff will develop their own palliative care plan to ensure the resident's comfort. This plan will include positive actions for the resident's benefit—special foods, music, massage, and con-sideration of a short trial of IV fluids and/or an appetite stimulant to improve his dehydration and resulting confusion.

DISCUSSION: Finish the session with further discussion about identi-fying when a nursing home resident is nearing death and appropriate actions for staff to take at that time.

ANNOTATED BIBLIOGRAPHY

Note to Facilitator: Before you present this session, if you would like to learn more about recognizing when death is approaching, we suggest the following articles.

Engle, V. F. (1998). Care of the living, care of the dying: Reconceptualizing nursing home care. *Journal of the American Geriatrics Society, 46,* 1172–1174.

This short but valuable commentary piece advocates hospice-type care for all permanently placed nursing home residents, including providing adequate symptom control, meeting spiritual needs, and helping residents remain in the nursing home until death. The author discusses barriers to providing this type of care and suggests changes needed in order for nursing homes to offer a holistic, integrated approach to comfort care.

Keay, T. J., & Schonwetter, R. S. (1998). Hospice care in the nursing home. *American Family Physician, 57,* 491–497.

This article describes the Medicare hospice benefit, discusses eligibility, and provides a table summarizing services available to nursing home residents enrolled in hospice programs. The article also includes a helpful "patient information handout" on hospice care in nursing homes, suitable for reproduction and distribution to residents and their families.

Long, M. C. (1996). Death and dying and recognizing approaching death. *Clinics in Geriatric Medicine, 12,* 359–367.

In this easily readable and informative work, Long covers many aspects of what we can expect as death approaches, including physical symptoms and mental and spiritual changes. She also discusses Elizabeth Kübler-Ross's stages of dying, writes about the concept of "appropriate death," and discusses grief and care for survivors.

Lynn, J. (2001). Serving patients who may die soon and their families: The role of hospice and other services. *JAMA, 285,* 925–932.

This article uses a case study to discuss both the benefits and the constraints of hospice programs. The author describes the three most common end-of-life trajectories: a short period of rapid decline, as with cancer; a long-term disability with an unpredictable timing of death, as with congestive heart failure; and an extended period of self-care deficits and a slowly dwindling course to death, as with dementia. She discusses the challenges in care planning for each of these trajectories, and advocates targeting for comprehensive end-of-life care those patients who "reasonably might die" within a year, rather than withholding these services for patients who "will die" within 6 months. This article also contains a one-page summary of guidelines for determining when a resident may be medically eligible for hospice services (reproduced in *Appendix A*) as well as a helpful list of text and Web-based resources.

Morrison, R. S., & Siu, A. L. (2000). Survival in end-state dementia following acute illness. *JAMA, 284,* 47–52.

This study looks at treatments and mortality rates for severely demented and cognitively intact patients hospitalized with hip fracture or pneumonia. For those with dementia and pneumonia, 6-month mortality was 53% and for those with dementia and hip fracture, 6-month mortality was 55%, compared with rates of 13% (pneumonia) and 12% (hip fracture) for the cognitively intact patients. Yet there was no difference by cognitive status with regard to use of "painful/ uncomfortable procedures," and, among the hip fracture group, patients with dementia received considerably less pain medication than did the cognitively intact patients.

Scheel, B. J., & Lynn, J. (1988). Care of dying patients. *Clinics in Geriatric Medicine, 4,* 639–654.

This article advocates that health care workers should attempt to attend to the physical, psychological, and personal needs of dying patients and their families, while recognizing the high levels of stress that families experience at these times. The authors, both physicians, comment on treatments for dealing with a range of symptoms commonly present at the end of life, including pain, anxiety, and depression, gastro-intestinal symptoms, urinary problems, skin breakdown, and respiratory problems.

3

Grief and Loss: Understanding and Supporting Families

> **Note to Facilitator:** Prior to this session, you should assemble a list of contacts for local grief, loss, and bereavement support services and bring a copy for each participant. Ask session participants to add to this list. *Time estimate: 60 minutes.*

OVERVIEW

This session addresses how nursing home staff can be most helpful to residents' family members and friends when death is approaching and grief reactions can be profound. The goal of this session is to provide you with practical tools you can use to help people in their grieving processes. Information from a recent study on death in nursing homes is included to give you concrete examples of concerns expressed by family members.

> **Instructions to Facilitator:** Present the following information to nursing home staff. Leave plenty of time for questions and discussion.

WHAT CAN WE LEARN FROM STUDIES OF FAMILIES WHO EXPERIENCE LOSS?

From 1998–2000, the authors of this training manual interviewed family members of recently deceased nursing home residents. The interviewers asked the family members about many aspects of care in the nursing home and about the quality of life experienced by their deceased family member in the last few months of her or his life. Some of the questions asked and a sample of family members' responses are printed below.

❐ What was one thing that helped your family member the most during the dying process?

- the presence and support of family, friends, and staff
- spiritual support from church friends
- staff attention to details of his care, to gentle touch, to listening
- being sedated so that she wasn't in pain
- normal pleasurable activities rather than a continual emphasis on death
- morphine

❐ Did your family member have a good death? If not, why not?

- too drawn out, too much suffering
- unresolved personal and spiritual conflicts
- no one to make decisions for him
- too long on life support
- lots of trouble breathing
- tremendous pain

❐ What was one thing that would have helped your family member during the dying process, but she or he did not receive?

- personal attention/care from staff, answering bell promptly, keeping her clean
- pain medication
- explanation of treatments or lack of treatments
- more visits from relatives

Note how different some of these items are, indicating the personal and individual nature of family and resident preferences. Also note how family concerns include physical, emotional, and spiritual needs.

FAMILY STRESSES DURING THE DYING PROCESS

❐ *Intense feelings* of sadness, anger, or guilt

❐ *Anticipatory mourning*, with conflict over whether to fight to hold on to a loved one or let them go

❐ *Uncertainty* about whether someone will live or die and about what type of medical treatment is right

❐ *Physical or cognitive changes* that make a dying family member unable to respond or make his appearance unfamiliar or upsetting

❐ *Stresses on family life* when it becomes a struggle to balance a dying person's needs with work demands and other relationships

❐ *Changes in family roles* when a grandparent, mother, or father is lost from family life and other members must take on new responsibilities at home

❐ *Practical issues* such as finances, wills, and funeral arrangements

❐ *Old family conflicts* that surface during times of crisis

❐ *Guilt* feelings over "abandoning" a loved one to a nursing home and uncertainty about how to be with a dying person

❐ *Concerns about quality of care* in the nursing home

DISCUSSION: Tell about a time that you were able to be particularly helpful to a family member of one of your residents. What did you do? Why was this helpful to your resident's family?

HELPING SOMEONE GRIEVE

The most important intervention you offer is *yourself.* You facilitate the grieving process by *being there,* by *listening,* and by offering your *presence* and *concern* more than advice. Here are some things you can do to help families with their grief:

❐ Remember that for you a resident's death is somewhat common, while for them it is a crisis.

❐ Encourage the saying of good-byes at the bedside before death, in whatever way is comfortable for family members.

❒ Show family members how to touch the dying resident, or even provide physical care such as mouth care, massage, or repositioning if they are comfortable doing so.

❒ Allow family members to bring personal mementos or special foods to the room, do laundry, or provide other types of personalized care.

❒ Encourage active participation in the care of the dying person, in being present at the moment of death, and even in preparing the body for burial if the family desires. Accept and do not judge family members who cannot bring themselves to participate in care or be present.

❒ Encourage involvement with the mourning rituals of funeral, eulogy, celebration, and memorial services.

❒ Listen without judging, and allow family members to voice concerns or tell stories. Encourage reminiscences, both painful and positive, and offer reassurance that mixed feelings are normal.

❒ Monitor your own feelings, realizing that you also may experience sadness or anxiety, and that you may want to express personal concern to the family.

❒ Be informed about support groups, hospice, and other bereavement programs in the area so you can refer family members who need help.

❒ Remind the family that you want to put the needs of the dying person first. Set clear limits when family conflicts appear to be harming or upsetting to the resident such as asking arguing persons to step out of hearing distance of the resident.

Instructions to Facilitator: After going through the material above, move on to the case-based example. Ask for a volunteer from the group to read the example and issues aloud, then pause for discussion and/or role-playing. Conclude the session by reading through and discussing the action plan and handing out homework.

An Example for Group Discussion

Case-Based Example: Ms. Wilson

Ms. Wilson, age 60, seems to the staff to be actively dying. She is a long-term resident of the facility who has end-stage kidney disease on hemodialysis and advanced dementia. Her chronic illnesses have resulted in immobility and dependence on tube feeding for all nutrition. She makes some eye contact with staff and family, but rarely communicates in words. Because she is incapable of decision-making, her son makes decisions for her. She has no advance directive and made no prior statements about her wishes for end-of-life care.

Over the past several months she has had repeated episodes of low blood pressure, resulting in incomplete dialysis and repeated trips to the ER without improvement. In recent weeks she has experienced episodes of pauses in her breathing.

Her son wishes his mother to go on living and feels that she is all he has. He is very attentive to her and has at times threatened to sue the nursing home when he feels her care is inadequate. He refuses a DNR order and wants "everything done" regarding treatment. Physicians at the hospital are frustrated by repeated ER visits by a dying resident and have asked that the nursing home not send this patient back to them. The nursing home physician is not responsive to this situation.

When she is clean and comfortable in her own bed, Ms. Wilson appears at peace. However, she experiences discomfort when turned or moved and appears distressed each time she is transported to the ER. Nursing home staff acknowledge that they do not know her wishes, but feel that her present treatment is cruel and doubt it to be in her best interest. They are deeply distressed by the possibility of their having to start CPR on this women and send her back to the ER to die in a strange place.

Issues to Consider

❐ *The staff feel they are at an impasse with the son, who is angry and grieving.*

❐ *Staff would like a way to authorize DNR and no further transfers to the hospital but feel helpless to change the present orders for her care.*

❐ *Ms. Wilson's prognosis is clearly terminal, yet staff doubt that her son has accepted this situation.*

STOP: Discuss the above case before going on to the action plan. What can staff do to ensure that Ms. Wilson has a good death? How can staff be most helpful to Ms. Wilson's son? Session participants may want to do a role play, acting out conversations between Ms. Wilson's son and various nursing home staff members.

An Action Plan for Ms. Wilson

❐ Staff plan to stop pushing the son for a DNR order, but instead work to acknowledge the son's deep and loving commitment to his mother. Their discussions with him will have a different focus—on the shared goals of her physical comfort, hygiene, and psychological peace. They will discuss a DNR order again only if they feel that these other aspects of care are well managed and sense that he feels the same.

❐ The son is likely to know his mother's prognosis, even if he is unable to admit it. Staff will stop saying "she is not doing well" and begin speaking directly about death by using the phrase "unfortunately, she seems to be dying." They will acknowledge their own sorrow at this loss, and ask the son how they can help him spend "special time" with his mother as she is dying.

❐ The physician will prescribe low-dose scheduled opioids to improve Ms. Wilson's physical comfort.

❐ Staff will acknowledge the son's grief and will provide support and emotional care.

❐ Staff will offer a referral to hospice and to a chaplain as a source of spiritual support for the son.

DISCUSSION: Finish the session with further discussion about working effectively with grieving family members.

ANNOTATED BIBLIOGRAPHY

Note to Facilitator: Before you present this session, if you would like to learn more about helping families cope with grief and loss, we suggest the following materials.

Bascom, P. B., & Tolle, S. W. (1995). Care of the family when the patient is dying, in Caring for Patients at the End of Life [special issue]. *Western Journal of Medicine, 163,* 292–296.

This article offers suggestions for communicating with families about a terminal diagnosis and discusses ways in which health care providers can give families support, guidance, and encouragement to begin planning for the decisions ahead. The authors state that providing high-quality care with excellent symptom control is one of the most comforting services that health care providers can offer to families. The authors also point out that extending an expression of sympathy, sending a condolence card, or making a follow-up phone call to a grieving relative after a death is often greatly appreciated by family members.

Churchill, L., Doron, M., Rothman, E., & Yarger, L. (2000). *Those Who Stay Behind: When a Family Member is Dying.* (31 minutes). Produced by VideoDialog. Distributed by Fanlight Productions, (800) 937-4113 or www.fanlight.com

This video presents interviews with five people who have recently lost family members. It is designed to be used with people in the midst of losing a family member and as a training tool for those who work with them. The accompanying Family Handbook includes both "Notes for Professionals" and "Notes for Families" outlining various ways to facilitate use of the video and issues to stimulate thinking and discussion. The video is divided into seven sections: Learning Bad News; Caretaking Decisions; Talking with Others; Taking Care of Each Other; Advance Directives and Later Decisions; Letting Go; and Those Who Stay Behind.

Krohn, B. (1998). When death is near: Helping families cope. *Geriatric Nursing, 19,* 276–278.

This short article discusses how to recognize grief responses in family members and how to respond with appropriate caring behaviors. This, in turn, will help families gain emotional control, complete unfinished business, work through anticipatory grief, and learn how to let go.

Wilson, S. A., & Daley, B. J. (November 1999). Family perspectives on dying in long-term care settings. *Journal of Gerontological Nursing, 25,* 19–25.

The authors interviewed family members who recently experienced the loss of a relative in a long-term care setting, asking the family members to discuss ways in which the staff had helped the family cope with their loss. Families commented that they were helped by staff who took the time to talk with them, to know the resident, and to listen to the families' concerns. Clearly explained advance directives, asking if families wanted to be present at the time of death, allowing families to express grief, and providing spiritual support (for example, praying with the residents and families) were also helpful to families in grief.

4

Advance Care Planning

Note to Facilitator: Prior to this session, prepare by learning the laws in your state on Living Wills, Health Care Powers of Attorney, use of feeding tubes, and other end-of-life treatment decisions. Bring in copies of advance directives that are legal in your state. Know the policies and procedures for documenting these things in the facility itself. *Time estimate: 90 minutes.*

OVERVIEW

Topics covered in this session include issues to consider in advance care planning, the Patient Self-Determination Act, staff involvement in the advance care planning process, outcomes of CPR, and decisions about whether to send a resident to the hospital. The objective of the session is to provide nursing home staff with knowledge and skills they can use to talk with residents and their families about goals of care and treatment choices.

Instructions to Facilitator: Lead nursing home staff through the following material, with time for questions and group discussions along the way.

WHAT IS ADVANCE CARE PLANNING?

❏ Advance care planning is the *process* of planning for one's final phase of life.

- ■ The discussion begins before a health crisis and should continue whenever residents, families, physicians, or staff have new concerns or a resident's health changes significantly

- ■ One staff member needs to take responsibility for facilitating the process within your nursing home: beginning the discussion, bringing advance care planning into care planning meetings, documenting resident preferences, and ensuring appropriate treatment orders

❏ Advance care planning includes:

- ■ introspection and discussion with one's family and health care providers

- ■ looking at values and priorities—what kind of health care matches my goals?

- ■ deciding what treatments one would want and not want if terminally ill, in a persistent vegetative state, or suffering from an incurable illness

- ■ choosing the care that would enhance quality of life and comfort

❏ Advance care planning in the nursing home should result in a plan of care to be used when a resident is in the final phase of her or his life.

- ■ The plan of care may include a DNR order but should not stop there

- ■ Planning should include discussion of hospitalization, tube feeding, and other treatment preferences

- ■ Planning should identify ways to enhance quality of life, bring emotional and spiritual support, and relieve pain and suffering

❏ An Advance Directives or Advance Care Planning section within each resident's medical chart is a good place to record information from all discussions with residents and families about their end-of-life care wishes. Having a designated section in each chart ensures that advance care planning wishes will be easy to find when they are needed and can be shared with all members of a resident's health care team. Photocopy this section of a resident's chart and make sure this information travels with a resident if she or he is transferred elsewhere.

WHO DECIDES—RESIDENT OR FAMILY?

❏ Try to include the resident as well as family members in all discussions; even residents with dementia or depression may have the capacity to express preferences and participate with family in the discussion.

❏ "Incompetence" is a legal term decided in a competency hearing, and it permanently removes decision-making authority from the individual to a surrogate.

- Formal competency assessment is rarely required to make end-of-life treatment decisions

- A person who is judged incompetent will also have a legally appointed guardian

❏ "Decisional capacity" is a *decision-specific* assessment made by a qualified clinician, usually a physician, who reviews whether the resident expresses consistent, coherent, and reasoned choices.

- The resident is assumed to be capable to make decisions

- A resident who lacks decisional capacity may still be included, with their family, in discussions of treatment decisions

- A health care power of attorney or a close family member can act as a surrogate decision-maker for residents who lack decisional capacity

❏ Some nursing home residents do not have family or are not emotionally close to anyone who could make hard decisions in their best interest. It is especially important for these residents to document their preferences in writing if possible. Alternatively, they may need a court-appointed guardian.

❏ Ethics committees, state ombudsman programs, or guardians-ad-litem may also provide consultation to facilitate decision making in the absence of a legal guardian or a natural family surrogate.

WHEN DO YOU START TALKING
ABOUT ADVANCE CARE PLANNING?

Talk to every new resident when she or he is admitted.

☐ The Patient Self-Determination Act of 1991 is a federal law requiring:

- that all residents be asked on admission if they have:

➤ a living will

➤ a health care power of attorney, legal proxy, or surrogate (not the same as power of attorney)

➤ any other kind of written advance directive

- that the answer to these questions be documented in medical records and communicated to health care staff

- that all residents be offered information on their right to make decisions concerning medical care and their right to create an advance directive

WHAT MIGHT YOU SAY IN A FIRST-TIME DISCUSSION?

☐ "We ask all patients if they have a living will or a health care power of attorney. Do you have these?"

- If yes, ask them to bring in forms. Ask who is the person named in the HCPOA and what is her/his phone number

- If no, offer information and provide forms and notary service to facilitate completion of written advance directives

- If a resident is uncomfortable completing legal forms, ask "Can you identify a person you would trust to make health care choices for you if you became unable to do this for yourself?"

☐ Reassure the resident or family member by saying "You don't have to decide anything right now. A doctor or nurse will discuss this more with you."

WHAT CAN YOU SAY TO RESIDENTS AND FAMILY MEMBERS?

☐ Begin the discussion by asking the resident and family what they know about the resident's health status. Gently clarify and correct any misunderstandings, and summarize what you know about the resident's health.

☐ Reassure by saying "We like to discuss with all residents what they want when their time comes, so we can honor their wishes. Can we talk about this now?"

☐ Ask about values and goals: "What makes life worth living now? What do you hope for now and in your future? What would make life *not* worth living?"

☐ "Where do you find strength in times of trouble? Do you have religious or spiritual beliefs that help you make tough decisions?"

☐ Ask "What do you hope doctors and nurses can do to help you (help your loved one)?"

☐ Ask "Who else would you turn to for help—family, friend, congregation, minister, rabbi?"

☐ Ask "Are there medical treatments that you fear or do not want?" If a family member must decide, say "Help us understand what your mother would want if she could speak to us now."

☐ Ask "Have you ever imagined what you would like your final hours or days of life to be like? Can you describe this?"

☐ Tell the resident: "We do not have to make all these decisions right now. We should talk about these issues again after you've had time to think it over and talk with your family."

☐ If the resident has a HCPOA, find out who that person is (name and how to reach him or her). Ask "Do they know your wishes?" and encourage discussion if the resident has not done so previously.

☐ If the resident doesn't have a health care power of attorney, ask "Who would you trust to speak for you if you were ill and couldn't make decisions?"

☐ If the resident has a living will, ask "What does that mean to you?"

☐ If the resident doesn't have a living will, ask "Do you (Did your father) have strong feelings about being on life support or heroic measures? What does 'heroic measures' mean to you (to him)?"

☐ Reassure resident of excellent comfort care. "We will always pay attention to your needs, and we promise to give you the best comfort care possible when you are dying."

END-OF-LIFE MEDICAL DECISIONS

This section briefly describes technological medical treatments and suggests some words you can use to discuss these issues with residents and families.

☐ "When death is approaching, there are some treatment choices. If you prefer a 'natural' death, you should express this wish and ask that treatments be used only to assure your comfort. Or you may want to try to live as long as possible, with the use of medical technology to prolong your life."

CARDIOPULMONARY RESUSCITATION (CPR)

☐ If the resident wants an attempt at CPR, clarify that this is a set of treatments to try to restart a person's heart and breathing at the moment of death. Let the resident know that for people in nursing homes, this procedure is rarely successful. For residents who survive a resuscitation attempt, there is no guarantee that they will recover their previous level of physical or mental functioning.
How many people survive CPR?

- In the hospital, for every 100 patients who receive a CPR attempt, 15 will survive

- In the nursing home, for every 100 residents who receive a CPR attempt, 2 to 5 will survive

- For patients over age 90, almost none will survive a CPR attempt

☐ "If your heart or breathing should stop, CPR can be attempted. In the nursing home, someone would do chest compressions and mouth-to-mouth resuscitation until emergency medical technicians arrive to place a breathing tube in your throat for assisted breathing. You will be taken to the hospital and attached to a ventilator. In most cases, CPR is not successful in reviving someone who is elderly or who is chronically or critically ill, and generally we do not recommend it."

VENTILATORS (BREATHING MACHINES)

A ventilator may prolong life temporarily, but the person must stay in an intensive care unit and will be sedated and unable to talk.

❏ If the resident wants a trial on a ventilator to see if survival is possible, ask how long this trial should last or if the resident would want to stay on life support indefinitely.

IV FLUIDS AND TUBE FEEDINGS

Most dying individuals want very little to eat or drink. This slowing-down process is normal and not painful. (Session 5, "Choices About Eating and Drinking," will aid your knowledge in this area.)

❏ Ask if the resident has wishes about IVs or tube feeding if terminally ill.

❏ Reassure that dehydration is not painful with comfort care.

HOSPITALIZATION DECISIONS

WHEN IS HOSPITALIZATION APPROPRIATE FOR A FRAIL NURSING HOME RESIDENT?

❏ To evaluate and diagnose treatable conditions and when function can be restored (for example, a heart attack in a person who is not terminally ill).

❏ To give treatment only available in the hospital (for example, to pin a hip fracture).

❏ To give comfort care not available in the nursing home (for example, a nerve block for pain).

WHEN IS HOSPITALIZATION INAPPROPRIATE FOR THAT SAME RESIDENT?

❏ When diagnosis and treatment can be done in the nursing home (for example, a urinary tract infection).

❏ When the burden outweighs the benefits (for example, IV antibiotics for a demented resident, who would have to be restrained and would be frightened by a strange place and unfamiliar people).

❏ When effective comfort care can be done in the nursing home— the resident's familiar environment.

HOW CAN NURSING HOME STAFF PARTICIPATE IN ADVANCE CARE PLANNING?

SOCIAL WORKER/ADMISSIONS OFFICER

☐ Begin discussion on admission, ask about advance directives.

☐ Educate residents and families about the choices they have. (See *Appendices C* and *D* for examples of ACP educational tools.)

CERTIFIED NURSING ASSISTANT

☐ You may be the first person to hear about a resident's fear of death, pain, or spiritual needs—allow the resident to talk, and offer comfort by listening.

☐ Reassure the resident that you will try to help her, or find others who can meet her needs.

☐ Report any comments about fears or treatment wishes to the nurse.

NURSE, NURSE PRACTITIONER, PHYSICIAN ASSISTANT, OR PHYSICIAN

☐ Discuss diagnosis, prognosis, goals of care, preferences, and treatment options—bring information to care planning.

☐ Chart this information in the Advance Directive or Advance Care Planning section of the resident's chart.

NURSE PRACTITIONER, PHYSICIAN ASSISTANT, OR PHYSICIAN

☐ Write medical orders such as "For comfort, liberalize diet to include all requested food or beverages," "Do not resuscitate," "Do not tube feed," or "Do not hospitalize." See *Appendix B* for suggestions regarding comfort care orders.

☐ Write order for hospice referral if resident or family desires this.

Instructions to Facilitator: After going through the material above, move on to the case-based example. Have someone in the group read the example and issues aloud, pausing for discussion along the way. Conclude the session by reading through and discussing the action plan and then handing out the homework for the week.

An Example for Group Discussion and Planning

Case-Based Example: Mr. Garrett

Mr. Garrett, a 65-year-old man, is admitted to the facility with severe terminal emphysema. His "responsible party" is a great-niece who cares for him but has not provided direct personal care during his illness. He suffers from mild to moderate dementia, and although he can talk, his ability to make decisions is unclear.

CPR was discussed with Mr. Garrett on admission, and he seemed unable to understand or make a consistent choice. He has since had several acute illnesses, and during one episode he asked the staff not to send him to the hospital. At present he is classified "full code" and is sent to the hospital every time he is acutely ill.

In the past one to two weeks Mr. Garrett has stopped eating and drinking and complains that he feels too tired and too short of breath to eat. He does not complain of any other discomfort but talks about heaven and has said good-bye to several favorite staff members.

Staff would like to ensure that Mr. Garrett has a peaceful death but fear that they will have to do CPR if he stops breathing. They believe hospice might be helpful.

Issues to Consider

❐   *What treatment decisions need to be discussed and clarified?*
❐   *How do you determine whether or not someone who has dementia can make decisions? What role does his great-niece have in medical treatment decisions? What can staff tell about his wishes from the statements he has made?*

☐ *Can hospice be called in, or can nursing home staff develop a comfort care plan?*

Instructions to Facilitator: Do one or more advance care planning role plays based on this case. For example, ask one staff member to pretend she is Mr. Garrett, one to pretend she is the great-niece, and one to be the nurse who begins a discussion of advance care planning, using some of the ideas from the section "*What can you say* . . . "Ask the participants to play their roles based on the ideal ways that residents, family members, and staff can discuss these hard issues.

DISCUSSION: How did it feel to be playing the role that you did? If you played the role of resident, did you find the advance care planning conversation helpful? Comforting? Frightening? Why? If you played the role of a staff person, were you comfortable discussing these issues with the resident? Why or why not? If you played the family member, what did you think was most important when decisions were made for Mr. Garrett?

Finish the session with further discussion about working with residents and their families to establish advance care plans.

ANNOTATED BIBLIOGRAPHY

Note to Facilitator: Before you present this session, if you would like to learn more about advance care planning, we suggest the following articles.

Ackerman, T. F. (1997). Forsaking the spirit for the letter of the law: Advance directives in nursing homes. *Journal of the American Geriatrics Society, 45,* 114–116. This editorial discusses findings from a study by Mezey, Mitty, Rappaport, and Ramsey (also in this issue of *JAGS*) designed to implement advance directives in a nursing home in New York City. Ackerman summarizes the difficulties that the study's authors encountered during their efforts to implement advance directives in the nursing home. Problems included advance directives completed by social workers without nurse or physician involvement; advance directives completed with residents but without involvement of proxies; a failure to review advance directives with residents at opportune times; and lack of portability of advance directives to alternative health care settings. Ackerman gives suggestions for ways in which nursing home professionals can address some of these concerns.

Crawley, L. M., Marshall, P. A., Lo, B., & Koenig, B. A. (2002). Strategies for culturally effective end-of-life care. *Annals of Internal Medicine, 136,* 673–679.

The authors assert that individual and cultural beliefs and values are of particular relevance at the end of life. When health care providers, patients, and families do not have a shared understanding of the meaning of illness or death, it can present challenges for agreeing on the best strategies to plan for the end of life or to alleviate pain and suffering. This paper offers suggestions for ways in which health care providers can assess the cultural background of each patient and inquire about values that may affect care at the end of life. Through developing "cultural sensitivity" and "cultural competence," health care providers can develop advance care planning processes that increase the possibility of comprehensive and compassionate end-of-life care.

Fischer, G. S., Arnold, R. M., & Tulsky, J. A. (2000). Talking to the older adult about advance directives. *Clinics in Geriatric Medicine, 16,* 239–254.

Fischer and colleagues present a case example of an elderly man who arrives in the emergency room in severe respiratory distress but with no advance directives, making treatment choices difficult. The authors then use this case to focus a discussion around how the issue might have been handled differently by the patient, his family, and his doctor prior to the patient's incapacitation. The authors offer clear and specific suggestions for communicating effectively with seniors about advance care planning.

Martin, D. K., Emanuel, L. L., & Singer, P. A. (2000). Planning for the end of life. *Lancet, 356,* 1672–1676.

In this paper the authors argue for a revised, patient-centered concept of advance care planning, moving away from a narrow focus on making treatment decisions in the event of incapacity and instead using the advance care planning process to help people "prepare for death." They assert that this process should include a focus on helping people achieve a sense of control, relieve burdens on loved ones, and strengthen or reach closure in relationships. They offer suggestions for advance care planning tools and approaches that can help patients achieve these goals.

Mezey, M. D., Mitty, E. L., Bottrell, M. M., Ramsey, G. C., & Fisher, T. (2000). Advance directives: Older adults with dementia. *Clinics in Geriatric Medicine, 16,* 255–268.

This article begins with an informative presentation about advance directives in general and then follows with a discussion of health care decision-making issues particularly relevant to persons with dementia. The article concludes by offering specific practice recommendations for working with individuals with dementia and their families to negotiate optimal treatment choices.

5

Choices About Eating and Drinking

> **Note to Facilitator:** Prior to this session, prepare by studying the laws of your state and the policy of your facility with regard to withholding or withdrawing feeding tubes or IV fluids. *Time estimate: 60 minutes.*

OVERVIEW

This session outlines the options for residents who have diminishing ability to nourish themselves. Some people see weight loss and dehydration as evidence of bad care in nursing homes. State surveyors and family members may blame nursing homes for these signs of declining health. However, decreased oral intake may also be a natural part of the dying process. This session reviews how stopping eating and drinking can be part of dying and is usually not uncomfortable. The session also discusses how to communicate with residents and families about treatment options and how to provide good comfort care. The goal of this session is for nursing home staff to be able to determine the best nutritional plans for residents' comfort while respecting residents' and families' wishes.

IS IT NORMAL FOR RESIDENTS WITH TERMINAL ILLNESS TO STOP EATING AND DRINKING?

❏ Two-thirds of terminally ill long-term care residents experience loss of appetite.

❏ Reduced need for nutritional intake is a normal part of the dying process, and most dying patients are not hungry or thirsty.

❏ Weight loss is expected in a dying resident; this is not painful and does not mean that the person is hungry. A dry mouth also occurs commonly in a dying resident. This should be treated with good mouth care. Although it is uncomfortable, a dry mouth does not mean that a person is thirsty.

WHAT HAPPENS WHEN A RESIDENT DOESN'T EAT OR DRINK?

❏ If residents stop eating but are still drinking fluids:

- they are able to live for weeks to months

- their feelings of hunger are blunted

- partial feeding may stimulate hunger

- their mental function may remain normal until just before death

❏ If residents stop drinking:

- they typically live one to three weeks but in rare cases may live as long as six weeks

- dehydration results in a gradual loss of consciousness

- death while dehydrated may be more peaceful and comfortable than death with IV fluids

- good mouth care is an important part of comfort care

WHAT GUIDANCE CAN WE OFFER TO RESIDENTS AND FAMILIES?

When nursing home residents stop eating or drinking, it is necessary to discuss their preferences for the use of tube feeding or IV fluids.

WHAT ARE SOME REASONS TO RECOMMEND USE OF TUBE FEEDING OR IV FLUIDS?

❏ Artificial nutrition and hydration can be used temporarily to support a resident who will recover from a nonterminal illness.

❐ These treatments may improve comfort for residents who express hunger or thirst.

❐ IV fluids may be used to keep a resident alert while awaiting a special visit or event prior to death. In this case, give fluids *temporarily* to treat delirium or loss of consciousness due to dehydration.

❐ Resident or family members' religious beliefs or strong feelings may require continued use of these treatments until death.

WHAT ARE REASONS NOT TO RECOMMEND TUBE FEEDING OR IV FLUIDS?

❐ Tube feedings and IV fluids can lead to increased lung secretions, shortness of breath, swelling, edema, and incontinence.

❐ Lack of IV fluids and tube feeding often results in a gradual, peaceful loss of consciousness.

❐ Artificial nutrition may prolong the dying process.

❐ Most dying residents do not experience hunger or thirst.

❐ Restraints may be necessary to hold IVs or feeding tubes in place, and this usually causes distress for residents and family members.

❐ Tube feeding does not provide taste pleasure or social contact around meals.

HOW DO WE MAKE GOOD DECISIONS ABOUT EATING AND DRINKING IN TERMINAL CARE?

❐ First evaluate the resident for treatable causes of reduced intake: depression, painful teeth, or other easily corrected problems.

❐ Consider a trial of an appetite stimulant, for example, methylphenidate 5 mg BID–10 mg TID or megestrol acetate 400–800 mg QD.

❐ Acknowledge the emotional and social meanings of food.

  ■ learn about and respect religious beliefs or cultural ideas that shape how a particular resident or family member deals with food

- recognize that, if a resident no longer wants or is unable to swallow fluids and food, families and nursing home staff lose an important way of feeling helpful to the resident

- suggest other comfort measures that they can use to help the dying resident, such as mouth care, positioning, massage, or music

- remember that natural loss of appetite and intake is not the same as "starving to death"

❐ Recognize the naturalness of stopping eating and drinking at the end of life.

- most dying patients are neither hungry nor thirsty

- fasting has been used for centuries to bring about religious experiences and spiritual preparedness

- dying "dry" may be more peaceful and comfortable, as IV fluids may cause discomfort from increased lung fluid, urinary incontinence, or vomiting

- when a person no longer wants or is unable to take in food or fluids, the body produces natural substances that enable a person to "drift away" comfortably

❐ Not imposing artificial nutrition and hydration is generally considered ethical in terminal illness.

- A few states have specific restrictions on decisions to withhold or withdraw these treatments—be sure you know the law in your state!

HOW DO WE PROVIDE GOOD MOUTH CARE?

Mouth care may be required every one to two hours or more frequently for an actively dying and highly dependent resident. Methods of care will depend on alertness of the resident, specific oral problems, and the response of the resident to mouth care.

❐ Assist with or perform regular toothbrushing with a small amount of toothpaste or mouthwash for more alert residents.

❐ Offer alcohol-free mouthwash to alert residents.

❐ Offer hard candies, ice chips, sips of water, favorite drinks, or water spray to residents who are alert. Be sure fluids are given with the resident sitting up, to prevent choking.

❐ Use chlorhexidine 0.12%, alcohol-free mouthwash, or water on swabs at regular intervals for less alert residents.

❐ Use hydrogen peroxide diluted 1:1 with water to remove crusting; do not use repeatedly. You may add a small amount of mint flavoring.

❐ Reduce medications causing dry mouth.

❐ Remove and clean dentures regularly.

❐ Treat thrush with topical antifungals, or a combination topical agent including an antifungal, viscous xylocaine, and diphenhydramine.

❐ Treat dry, cracked lips with petroleum jelly, lip balm, or ointment with vitamins A&D.

❐ If a resident shows distress during mouth care, such as shaking her head, do not insist on it. Try a small ice chip in the front of her mouth or cheek.

Instructions to Facilitator: After going through the material above, move on to the case-based example. Have someone in the group read the example and issues aloud, then pause for discussion. Conclude the session by reading through and discussing the action plan and then handing out the homework for the session.

An Example for Group Discussion and Planning

Case-Based Example: Mr. Murphy & Ms. Lewis

Mr. Murphy is a 79-year-old man with terminal lung cancer. He has a chronic productive cough and shortness of breath, but receives oxygen and regular morphine with good control of these symptoms. He has lived in the nursing home for several months, after his physical weakness made it difficult for him to live at home. His family visits often, and they are very supportive.

Mr. Murphy is slowly but steadily losing weight. He seems to find it difficult to eat a full meal, in part because he becomes fatigued while eating. He has had one episode of dehydration with pneumonia, which was treated with IV fluids and antibiotics. Because of his steady weight loss and poor intake, his doctor, nurse, and aide discuss choices about eating and drinking with the resident and his family. Their initial reaction is one of concern: they want any treatment that will improve his energy and rebuild his strength, though everyone recognizes he is dying of cancer.

Another resident in the nursing home, Ms. Lewis, has advanced Alzheimer's disease and has developed poor intake of food and water. She swallows fairly well, but shows little interest in food or drink and has to be encouraged to take each bite. She is physically fairly inactive, but is still losing weight at the rate of 20 pounds over the past 3 months. Since the patient lacks decision-making capacity and never mentioned tube feeding in her living will, her doctor, nurse, and aide discuss how to approach her family with treatment options for this problem.

Issues to Consider

☐ *Mr. Murphy has little appetite and expresses no hunger, and he and his family understand that he is terminally ill.*

☐ *Ms. Lewis has end-stage dementia, but her family may not have acknowledged this.*

☐ *Mr. Murphy is able to participate in discussions about his treatment options and to make his wishes known.*

☐ *Ms. Lewis does not have decision-making capacity and has no written directives outlining her thoughts about artificial nutrition.*

STOP: Compare the above cases before going on to the action plan. What would you recommend for Mr. Murphy and Ms. Lewis?

An Action Plan for Mr. Murphy and Ms. Lewis

❏ Assess both residents for reversible causes of their lack of intake and weight loss (for example, check for thyroid disease, dental or mouth pain, drug effects, depression).

❏ Liberalize their diets with soft and chewable but appealing foods. Encourage them to eat anything they especially like.

❏ Increase staff time to assist with meals of favorite foods.

❏ Discuss appetite stimulants (methylphenidate or megestrol acetate) with physician and resident/family.

❏ Provide careful mouth care.

❏ Involve the family as caregivers, suggesting non-food-oriented ways that they can offer their family member comfort, such as encouraging them to provide mouth care.

❏ Counsel Mr. Murphy, his family, and Ms. Lewis's family about treatment options, letting them know that lack of intake is not painful or uncomfortable.

❏ Let Mr. Murphy and his family know that not using artificial nutrition may decrease his secretions and improve his shortness of breath.

❏ Support family decision making, offering reassurance that not using artificial nutrition will not cause suffering.

DISCUSSION: Finish the session with further discussion about helping residents and families to make choices about eating and drinking.

ANNOTATED BIBLIOGRAPHY

Note to Facilitator: Before you present this session, if you would like to learn more about making choices about eating and drinking near the end of life, we suggest the following articles.

Byock, I. R. (1995). Patient refusal of nutrition and hydration: Walking the ever finer line. *American Journal of Hospice & Palliative Care, 12,* 8–13. (Also available online at www.dyingwell.org/prnh.htm)

Byock presents summaries of multiple studies of the effects of fasting and dehydration in individuals near the end of life. He also comments thoughtfully on a number of the ethical and clinical issues involved in these decisions.

Jackonen, S. (July-September 1997). Dehydration and hydration in the terminally ill: Care considerations. *Nursing Forum, 32*, 5–13.

This article is a review of the literature on terminal dehydration. It defines terminal dehydration, discusses the benefits and disadvantages of withholding medical hydration and nutrition, and offers suggestions for research and practice.

Mitchell, S. L., Tetroe, J., & O'Connor, A. M. (2001). A decision aid for long-term tube feeding in cognitively impaired older persons. *Journal of the American Geriatrics Society, 49*, 313–316.

The authors describe the development and evaluation of a decision aid to be used by substitute decision makers in an acute-care hospital. The aid significantly increased decision makers' knowledge and decreased their decisional conflict. All decision makers also reported that they found the aid to be helpful and acceptable, despite the difficult and emotional circumstances they faced.

Parkash, R., & Burge, F. (Winter 1997). The family's perspective on issues of hydration in terminal care. *Journal of Palliative Care, 13*, 23–27.

This article outlines the concerns of family members around the issue of terminal dehydration. Issues discussed include fear of prolongation of dying by using artificial fluids as well as increased suffering without fluids. Diverse factors influenced families' decision-making processes. The article highlights the importance of education and open discussion between health care professionals and patients and their families.

Printz, L. A. (1992). Terminal dehydration: A compassionate treatment. *Archives of Internal Medicine, 152*, 697–700.

This paper argues that once comfort has been chosen as the goal of care, medical hydration and nutrition are no longer appropriate in most cases. The author uses three short case studies to illustrate his point. He discusses the effects of terminal dehydration and offers suggestions for ways other than giving food and drink that medical professionals can show care and compassion for their patients.

Smith, S. A., & Andrews, M. (2000). Artificial nutrition and hydration at the end of life. *MEDSURG Nursing, 9*, 233–244.

This article is designed for nurses and other health care professionals who care for and educate patients regarding IV fluids and tube feedings. It discusses some of the ethical, religious, and legal opinions regarding this topic. The authors provide two useful tables with simple suggestions for making food intake as comfortable as possible (for example, "offer small servings on small plates and serve more frequently" and "to conserve energy and/or reduce frustration, use 'sippy cups' or large straws"). They also include helpful information that can be shared with family members regarding nutritional needs at the end of life, and they discuss ways to refocus caring emotions to provide "nourishment" to dying individuals in ways other than through food or fluids. They conclude, "The patient's mind and spirit can be nourished with genuine and loving words and gestures, pain control, intellectual stimulation, spiritual guidance, and humor. In this way, the goal of comfort will be achieved."

Zerwekh, J. V. (March 1997). Do dying patients really need IV fluids? *American Journal of Nursing, 97*, 26–31.

This article, written by a hospice nurse, offers a thorough discussion of the benefits and burdens of IV fluids. The author lists numerous ways in which IV fluids might add to the discomfort of a dying individual, as well as discussing circumstances in which IV fluids would be beneficial. She also offers helpful and specific guidelines about how to discuss this difficult issue with physicians, other members of the care team, and family members.

6

Pain Management

Notes to Facilitator: Although this session may be presented to a mixed audience, the needs of nurses and CNAs are different, so separate educational sessions are recommended. This session includes some materials relevant primarily to licensed nursing staff and other materials relevant primarily to CNAs, social workers, and other staff who do not administer medications. *Time estimate: 90 minutes.*

OVERVIEW

This session discusses assessing and treating pain in terminally ill nursing home residents. This session assumes that:

(1)   a good care plan can almost always alleviate pain,
(2)   every member of the care team has a responsibility to participate in pain management,
(3)   it is impossible to have high-quality end-of-life care when a resident is in pain
(4)   people facing death have a profound fear of being in pain.

The goal of this session is for staff to recognize when residents are experiencing pain and to know how to assess pain and respond appropriately until a resident is comfortable.

> **Instructions to Facilitator:** Lead nursing home staff through the following material, with time for questions and group discussions along the way, particularly as indicated in the text.

DEFINITION OF PAIN

❐ "Pain is whatever the person experiencing it says it is, and it exists whenever the person says it does."
—Margo McCaffery, nurse and pain management expert

❐ Pain may be expressed by changes in usual behavior—especially in residents with dementia. They may become *more* distressed and agitated or *less* active and more withdrawn from normal interactions and activities.

❐ Older patients may be stoic and unwilling to admit to feeling pain—asking about "discomfort" may be more useful than asking about "pain."

PAIN AMONG NURSING HOME RESIDENTS

❐ 45–80% of nursing home residents have pain

❐ One out of two *dying* residents have moderate to severe pain

❐ The most common causes of pain are cancer and arthritis resulting in bone and nerve pain

❐ One out of four residents with *daily pain* receives *no* medication for pain

MANY NURSING HOME RESIDENTS HAVE CHRONIC PAIN

Acute pain is easier to recognize than chronic pain—nursing home staff need to be able to recognize and treat both types of pain.

Acute Pain	**Chronic Pain**
(Examples: broken bone, sudden abdominal pain)	*(Examples: arthritis, tooth decay, osteoporosis)*
Recent onset, change	Long-standing
New pain complaint	Old or no complaint
Anxiety, grimacing, restless movement	Mood depressed, withdrawn, listless
Increased pulse and BP, muscle tension, sweating	No change in vital signs, may not appear to be in pain

WHAT ARE THE BARRIERS TO TREATING PAIN?

❐ The myth that pain is to be expected and that pain cannot be managed

❐ Resident Factors:

- belief that pain is part of normal aging
- concern that it is not acceptable to show pain or to take medications for pain
- dementia and speech problems make it difficult to describe pain

❐ Caregiver Factors:

- belief that older patients feel less pain than younger patients
- difficulty recognizing chronic pain
- belief than pain is part of normal aging
- idea that elders cannot tolerate opioid medication
- fear of addiction or overdose

❐ System Factors:

- lack of easily accessible pain medications
- inadequate staff education about pain management
- inadequate numbers of staff to assess and treat pain in all residents

❐ Most common barrier is caregiver **failure to ask and assess pain**

HOW DO YOU KNOW IF A RESIDENT HAS PAIN?

☐ **Ask every resident routinely** if she or he has any pain or discomfort. For example, ask, "Have you had any pain today?" "Have you had any discomfort today?" "Are you uncomfortable right now?" "Are you hurting right now?" For a resident with suspected or known pain, ask more frequently until pain is controlled.

☐ **Find out how severe a resident's pain is on the pain scale used in your facility**—remember residents' glasses or hearing aids if needed! Two sample pain scales are attached below. See *Appendix B* for more examples of pain scales.

Example 1: Verbal Pain Scale

Ask the resident: "On a scale of 0 to 10, with 0 being no pain, 1–3 being mild pain, 4–6 being moderate pain, and 7–10 being severe pain, with 10 being the worst pain you can imagine, what number would you say best describes your pain right now?"

0:	No Pain
1–3:	Mild Pain
4–6:	Moderate Pain
7–10:	Severe Pain

Example 2: Faces Scale

Say to the resident: "There are six faces below. The first face is a smiling, happy face, meaning no pain. The last face is a sad, crying face, meaning severe pain. The four middle faces are somewhere in between. Point to or draw a mark beside the face that best describes your pain right now."

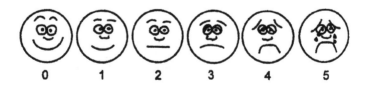

☐ **Also ask about location, quality, and duration of pain**—"What worsens or relieves the pain?"

❐ **Observe resident**—what non-verbal cues may indicate pain?

- Decrease in self-care

- Changes in vital signs

- Expressions of distress or withdrawal

- Changes in behavior, including increased restlessness, agitation, aggression, or unusual withdrawal or stillness

❐ Review diagnoses—could any of them be causing pain?

HOW CAN YOU ASSESS PAIN IN RESIDENTS WITH DEMENTIA?

❐ Remember that the best indicator that a cognitively impaired resident is in pain is a *change in behavior.*

❐ In addition to observation of residents, **ask them**—four out of five residents with dementia can report pain if asked.

❐ You may need different pain scales for residents with dementia. Three sample pain scales that work particularly well for people with dementia are attached below. See *Appendix B* for more examples of pain scales.

**Example 3: Verbal Pain Scale
(Present Pain Intensity Scale)**

Ask the resident: "On a scale of 0 to 5, with 0 being no pain, 1 being mild pain, 2 being discomforting pain, 3 being distressing pain, 4 being horrible pain, and 5 being excruciating pain, what number would you say best describes your pain right now?"

    0 — No Pain
    1 — Mild Pain
    2 — Discomforting Pain
    3 — Distressing Pain
    4 — Horrible Pain
    5 — Excruciating Pain

Example 4: Color Pain Scale

Say to the resident: "The line below represents "no pain" at one end and "worst possible pain" at the other end. Point to or draw a mark on the point on the line that best describes your pain right now."

Example 5: Simple Verbal Pain Scale

Say to the resident, "Do you have any pain [or discomfort] *right now?*" If they indicate yes, then ask, "Is your pain [or discomfort] mild, moderate, or severe?"

No Pain	Mild Pain	Moderate Pain	Severe Pain

Note that you ask about pain *right now.* People with dementia might not remember if they had pain at an earlier time.

Note that you ask only "mild, moderate, or severe," without asking the resident to give a number.

❏ It is particularly important to look for changes in:

- breathing (noisy, labored, or rapid)

- vocalizations (crying out; moaning; change in pitch, pattern, or volume)

- facial expressions (sad or frightened expression, grimacing, tears, eyes narrowed or unfocused, wrinkling of forehead when moved)

- behavior (fidgeting, restlessness, crying, tense rocking, rubbing or holding a body part, aggression, resistance to movement or personal care, agitation)

Information for Licensed Nursing Staff

> **Note to Facilitator:** The following sections (on types of pain and pain medications) are useful primarily to licensed nursing staff. Adjust the amount of time you spend on these topics depending on your particular audience.

WHAT ARE DIFFERENT TYPES OF PAIN AND THEIR CAUSES?

❐ *Somatic:* localized tissue destruction (Examples: bone pain, pain after surgery or trauma)

❐ *Visceral:* stretching internal organs (Examples: bowel obstruction, angina, urinary retention, constipation)

❐ *Neuropathic:* injury to nerves (Examples: diabetic foot pain, pinched nerve, shingles)

- Knowing the kind of pain a resident has will influence medication choices

- Whenever possible, treat the underlying cause of pain; for example, for visceral pain caused by a stool impaction, relieve the impaction

WHAT ARE ELEMENTS OF A COMPLETE PAIN ASSESSMENT?

❐ Know why a resident may have pain

- diagnoses that predispose to pain (e.g., arthritis)

- progression of a disease (e.g., cancer)

- acute problem (e.g., hairline hip fracture, urinary retention)

❐ Know the specifics of a resident's pain

- character (e.g., dull, sharp, burning, aching, radiating)

- location

- intensity

- timing (e.g., onset, duration, time of day when worst)

- factors that aggravate

- factors that relieve

- associated symptoms (e.g., nausea, vomiting)

- effect on function

- physical assessment of the site of pain

- history of pain and coping mechanisms used in the past

❏ Know the specifics of a resident's treatment

  - pain medications currently taking (including dosage and schedule)

  - PRN medications given

  - complimentary therapies given

WHAT ARE IMPORTANT ISSUES IN MEDICATION USE?

After you find that a resident is in pain, the next step is to call the prescriber. Be prepared to report vital signs, the severity of pain, the medications that have already been tried and their effectiveness. Know the best way to use pain medications:

❏ Scheduled dosing, not PRN

❏ Begin with a short-acting medication. Once it works well, change to a *long-acting* scheduled medication with a *short-acting* PRN medication for breakthrough pain

❏ Assess response

  - 15–30 minutes after IV

  - 30–60 minutes after PO or rectal administration

  - 2–3 days after patch (with concurrent administration and assessment of a short-acting agent for breakthrough pain)

❏ Keep increasing dose and/or frequency until desired effect is achieved or until resident experiences side effects

❐ Give dose before pain becomes severe

❐ Bowel regimen starts when opioids start

❐ Consult your pharmacist or an equianalgesic pain medication table (see *Appendix B* for an example) for typical dosing schedules.

❐ Provide feedback to CNAs regarding changes in the resident's treatment plan. Encourage CNAs to continue to report any signs of pain or discomfort they observe while at the resident's bedside.

❐ Document and communicate across disciplines and across shifts.

❐ Use complementary (nonpharmacologic) therapies for pain relief in addition to medication.

Information for CNAs and Other Staff Who Provide Comfort Care

> **Note to Facilitator:** The following sections (on comfort measures, relaxation exercises, and the special role of CNAs) should be particularly useful for CNAs, activities directors, social workers, recreation therapists, and volunteers. Adjust the amount of time you spend on these topics depending on your particular audience.

CNAs are often the people most likely to notice when a resident is acting differently or showing subtle signs of pain, since these extremely valuable staff members are the ones most often at the bedside. CNAs, therefore, play a crucial role in pain identification and relief. CNAs should take an active approach to helping residents with pain, reporting their observations to the nurses regularly and providing comfort measures to residents as often as possible.

WHAT COMFORT MEASURES CAN *YOU* PROVIDE?

❐ Supportive talk and gentle touch

❐ Music, soft lighting, decreased noise

❐ Warm or cold packs according to nurse's instructions

❐ Massage and repositioning

❏ Gentle movement, self-care assistance, or time out of bed—find the level of activity that brings the most comfort to the resident

❏ Prayer and spiritual support, conversation and listening

❏ A favorite drink or food

❏ Help with personal cleanliness—bed bath, full bath, mouth care

❏ Reminiscing with the resident about a favorite time in her life, or favorite hobby, or special times with her family

❏ A walk

❏ Helping the resident find something of interest that distracts him from his pain: singing, reading the Bible, watching TV, humor

WHAT ARE SOME SPECIAL RELAXATION EXERCISES THAT YOU CAN OFFER TO RESIDENTS?

❏ Create a calm atmosphere, then slowly say to the resident, pausing between each suggestion: "Close your eyes and take a deep breath. Let go of any worries. Imagine that you are at your favorite place—maybe the mountains or the beach or the woods. As you relax in your chair or hammock, imagine all the sights around you, the sounds around you, the smells. Imagine that you have all the time in the world to enjoy this pleasant spot."

❏ Before starting, ask the resident to tell you a word, phrase, or scene that brings her pleasure or comfort (for example, "peace," "calm," or "the Lord is my Shepherd"). Then ask her if there is a word that expresses something she wants to get rid of (for example, "stress," "fear," or "pain"). Instruct the resident: "Close your eyes and take a deep breath. Think of the special word or phrase that brings you pleasure and comfort. Focus on this word or phrase every time you breathe in. Every time you breathe out, think of the word or phrase that you want to release. Imagine blowing it away with each breath as you exhale."

DISCUSSION: What comfort measures that you have provided to residents or loved ones in the past have been especially helpful in managing pain and providing relief?

REMEMBER THE SPECIAL ROLE CNAS PLAY IN PAIN RELIEF

❏ Ask your residents, "Where does it hurt? What makes it better? What makes it worse?"

- You should ask about both pain and discomfort

- Use the same pain scale the nurse is using and one that you and the resident agree works for the resident

- For residents unable to speak, look for changes in behavior

☐ Report what you know about a resident's pain to the nurse

- You may well be the first one who knows a resident is in pain—alert others

- You will often be the first one who knows whether treatment works or does not help—let the nurse know

- You can use your skills in personal care and your relationship with the resident to help her to relax, find comfortable positions, and find distractions from pain

☐ CNAs and nurses need to work as a team to control pain—both of you have important roles

- You can observe what helps and what hurts—report your ideas to the nurse

Information for All Nursing Home Staff

Note to Facilitator: The following summary of pain management issues should be presented to all nursing home staff.

REMEMBER EACH OF THESE STEPS
FOR SUCCESSFUL PAIN MANAGEMENT

☐ Assessment of pain and discomfort—document using pain scale

☐ Remember the valuable role that CNAs play in pain relief, since they are the staff members most often at the bedside and most likely to notice changes in behavior and other subtle signs of pain

☐ Review of treatment history and current medication use

☐ Development and implementation of medication schedule and nonmedical treatments to relieve pain—document in care plan

❐ Reassessment of pain and discomfort and effectiveness of treatments used

❐ Adjustment of treatment plan

❐ Pain management requires whole team

- *CNA:* observes, reports evidence of pain to nurse, gives comfort measures, observes response of resident to medication and pain relief strategies and reports to nurse

- *Nurse:* assesses, treats, and reassesses pain; continues refinement of treatment until resident obtains relief; provides feedback to CNAs about changes made in treatment plans

- *MD/NP/PA:* diagnoses causes of pain and orders medications or other treatments

- *Hospice or palliative care consultant:* Hospice provides added expert help with pain management for dying nursing home residents

❐ High-quality care for pain requires continuous assessment, adjustment of treatment, reassessment, communication, and documentation.

Instructions to Facilitator: After going through the material above, move on to the case-based example. Have someone in the group read the example and issues aloud, then pause for discussion. Conclude the session by reading through and discussing the action plan and then handing out the homework for the session.

An Example for Group Discussion and Planning

Case-Based Example: Ms. Miller

An elderly woman, Ms. Miller, has been diagnosed with lung cancer. After some time, her disease spreads to her neck, which causes difficulty swallowing. She has mild dementia but can make her own care decisions. She also suffers from chronic back pain, which has now become more severe.

Facility staff have known her for years. She loves classical music and is deeply religious. She had an abusive marriage and tends to not talk about her own needs and avoids disturbing others. Staff describe her personality as very passive. Ms. Miller never says she is in pain and avoids answering a direct question such as "Are you feeling any pain now?"

Nurses who know Ms. Miller observe she is less physically active than in past months. She is less willing to move from her bed to a chair and appears tired and withdrawn when they try to talk with her. Aides have reported she grimaces during bathing but responds well to gentle touch. These observations lead staff to agree that she is experiencing daily physical pain.

She has a DNR order, and the hospice team is providing additional palliative care and spiritual and emotional support. She has taken Percocet for back pain in the past but has recently received long-acting oxycodone (Oxycontin) 30 mg PO BID plus oxycodone 10 mg every 4 hours for breakthrough pain. This still does not seem to be enough.

Issues to Consider

☐ How can staff assess pain, given that the resident doesn't like to complain and that she has mild dementia?

☐ What behaviors and expressions make CNAs and other staff think that Ms. Miller is in pain?

☐ Pain management needs to be improved, and staff would like to change all medication to nonoral forms because of her difficulty swallowing.

☐ What comfort measures can staff use to help relieve Ms. Miller's pain?

☐ How will staff know when Ms. Miller's pain is relieved?

STOP: Discuss and design a care plan for the team to treat Ms. Miller's pain.

An Action Plan for Ms. Miller

☐ A primary nurse is assigned who has won the trust of this resident. She tests several pain scales. A visual color-coded scale appears to work best, because it allows Ms. Miller to point and to avoid using the word "pain." All other staff agree to use this scale.

☐ The primary nurse contacts the physician and discusses the need for nonoral pain medication. She reports that Ms. Miller uses a total of 120 mg of oxycodone per day, equivalent to 180 mg of morphine. They discuss other options, and the physician tapers oral oxycodone and orders fentanyl 75 mcg patch q72 hours with concentrated liquid morphine 10 mg q2 hours as needed for breakthrough pain.

☐ Nurses let the CNAs know that they all are working together to relieve Ms. Miller's pain.

☐ Family members and nursing home volunteers agree to spend extra time with Ms. Miller to talk and play tapes of her favorite hymns.

☐ CNAs on every shift clean Ms. Miller's dry mouth with swabs moistened with water and apply moisturizer to her lips.

☐ CNAs offer to read the Bible or pray with her if they feel comfortable.

☐ After obtaining Ms. Miller's permission, the social worker notifies the resident's pastor about her condition, and he visits. Ms. Miller also continues to receive supportive visits from the hospice chaplain.

☐ When CNAs go off shift, they pass on information to the new staff members about comfortable repositioning and the gentle touch that seems to help Ms. Miller.

DISCUSSION: Finish the session with further discussion about pain management.

ANNOTATED BIBLIOGRAPHY

Note to Facilitator: Before you present this session, if you would like to learn more about pain management, we suggest the following materials.

Acello, B. (April 2001). Focus on pain: The nurse assistant's role in pain management. *Journal of Nurse Assistants,* 18–32.
   This article contains a multitude of user-friendly suggestions and helpful materials that nursing assistants could use in the workplace on a daily basis. The article highlights the JCAHO pain standards, discusses barriers to effective pain management, lists nonverbal signs and symptoms that can indicate pain, and provides examples of a variety of pain scales. This journal offers special group rates to nursing homes, as well as a 30 percent discount when they send 10 or more copies of the magazine to the same address. For ordering information, call (440) 247-5668 or write PO Box 23365; Chagrin Falls, OH 44023.

American Geriatrics Society Panel on Persistent Pain in Older Persons (2002). The management of persistent pain in older persons. *Journal of the American Geriatrics Society, 50,* S205–S224.
   This paper offers specific recommendations for assessing pain, treating pain with pharmacologic approaches, treating pain with nonpharmacologic strategies, and modifying health care systems to provide greater pain management. The article also contains numerous useful charts and tables, including pain scales; assessment forms; and lists of medications, dosages, precautions, and recommendations.

Medical College of Wisconsin (2000). *Nursing Staff Education Resource Manual: Pain Management 101.* Available from Medical College of Wisconsin Research Foundation, Inc. To order, contact the Palliative Care Program, Division of Hematology/ Oncology, Medical College of Wisconsin, 9200 W. Wisconsin Ave., Milwaukee, WI 53226-3596, telephone (414) 805-4605.
   This manual offers a six-session in-service education program in pain management for long-term care facilities. Topics include assessing pain, medication issues, nonpharmacological interventions, assessing discomfort in patients with dementia, and communicating with doctors about a resident's pain. The manual also includes a disk with handouts and Power Point slides for presenting the material in a group setting.

Medical College of Wisconsin (1998). *Improving Pain Management in Long-Term Care Settings: A Resource Guide for Institutional Change.* Available from Medical College of Wisconsin Research Foundation, Inc. To order, contact the Palliative Care Program, Division of Hematology/Oncology, Medical College of Wisconsin, 9200 W. Wisconsin Ave., Milwaukee, WI 53226-3596, telephone (414) 805-4607.
   This "how to" resource manual is designed to assist staff members of long-term care facilities to develop systemic methods of improving pain assessment and management in their facilities. The manual provides examples of institutional philosophy statements concerning pain, pain assessment tools, pain policies and

procedures, educational outlines, and other useful information and forms that nursing homes can use as is, or take as a starting point and adapt to meet their specific needs.

Seskevich, J. (2000). Video: *Guided Relaxation with Touch Therapy* (43 minutes). Durham, NC: Stress Management Education. To order, go to www.managestress now.com or call (919) 286-1207.

This affordable videotape offers simple, clear instructions on helping others with stress and pain management. It includes a variety of specific interactions that all health care practitioners can incorporate into their everyday practice.

Stein, W. M., & Ferrell, B. A. (1996). Pain in the nursing home. *Clinics in Geriatric Medicine, 12,* 601–613.

This paper provides an overview of pain in nursing homes, offering a description of the scope of the problem, discussing the barriers to pain management in long-term care settings, and then highlighting reasons why nursing homes have the potential to manage pain well, given their unique interdisciplinary approach to care planning and provision. The article discusses pain assessment, including presenting several pain scales, and then offers advice for pain treatment, with specific suggestions for dealing with musculoskeletal, neuropathic, and malignant pain, as well as mild, moderate, and severe pain.

Whitecar, P. S., Jonas, A. P., & Clasen, M. E. (2000). Managing pain in the dying patient. *American Family Physician, 61,* 755–764.

These authors assert that with appropriate assessment and use of analgesics, health care professionals should achieve successful pain relief for over 90 percent of dying patients. The authors discuss the use of corticosteroids, antidepressants, and anticonvulsants, as well as narcotics, for pain management. They also offer suggestions for anticipating and treating side effects of medications, and they advocate a team approach to pain management.

7

Emotional and Spiritual Care

OVERVIEW

One purpose of this session is to understand the ways in which dying is much more than the death of a body. Dying and death are profound human, social, and spiritual events. Presented below are some of the emotional and spiritual concerns that individuals encounter as death draws near, along with suggestions about how we as caregivers can help our residents, not only by addressing their physical needs, but also by ministering to their emotional and spiritual needs. Remember, however, that not everyone wants to talk about death in emotional and spiritual terms. **The ministry of presence is the most powerful comfort you can offer.**

> **Instructions to Facilitator:** Lead nursing home staff through the following material, with time for questions and group discussions along the way. Remind participants that they can only work effectively with emotional and spiritual needs if they reflect on their own emotional state and religious beliefs and can distinguish between their needs and their residents' needs. Note that a section of this module is relevant primarily to licensed nursing staff and medical prescribers. *Time estimate: 60 minutes.*

WHAT ARE SOME OF THE EMOTIONAL CONCERNS OF INDIVIDUALS NEAR THE END OF LIFE?

❏   How will I die?

❏   Will it be painful?

❐ Will I get the care I need?

❐ Will I be alone?

❐ Am I a burden on my family?

❐ Will I lose my ability to control what happens to me? If I do, who will be in control?

❐ What will happen to my family if I die?

❐ Are there things I need or want to say to family and friends before I die?

WHAT ARE SOME OF THE SPIRITUAL CONCERNS OF INDIVIDUALS NEAR THE END OF LIFE?

❐ Why am I dying?

❐ Where will I go after death?

. ❐ What was meaningful about my life?

❐ What meaning can I find in my dying?

❐ What can I do to be spiritually ready for my death?

WHAT CAN WE LEARN FROM STUDIES OF THE EMOTIONAL NEEDS OF PEOPLE FACING DEATH?

❐ **Emotional Stages of Dying:** Dr. Elizabeth Kübler-Ross interviewed many cancer patients who were terminally ill, and they often experienced the emotional reactions listed below. It may be difficult or impossible for residents with advanced dementia to experience these stages. Most dying patients do not proceed through all these stages in a defined order:

■ *denial*—the resident cannot accept she/he is dying

■ *anger*—can also be expressed as fear, resentment, frustration, and a struggle with the emotional and spiritual questions related to death

■ *bargaining*—trying to "make a deal" with God in order to avoid death or suffering

- *depression*—can be grief over past losses, disappointments, and unfulfilled dreams, or preparation for death; may also be expressed as withdrawal, detachment

- *acceptance*—can lead to a time of calm and peacefulness

❑ **Interviews With Terminally Ill Nursing Home Residents:** Dr. Veronica Engle interviewed dying nursing home residents and found their experiences and their emotional and social concerns to be somewhat different from Kübler-Ross's traditional stages of dying:

- *the living-dying interval*—Many residents have a long period of time between the knowledge that they will die from the chronic illnesses that brought them to the nursing home, and the experience of active dying

- *residents focused on the quality of their day-to-day living*—When death is near, time becomes very precious; there is a need to enhance the quality of life moment by moment. Residents wanted to experience many of the ordinary pleasures of life and relationships, without a constant focus on dying.

- *racial and cultural differences*—African-Americans sometimes receive less pain control and poorer comfort care. Minority residents may need special attention to improve their care.

DISCUSSION: What are some of the emotional and spiritual concerns that residents tell you about or that you observe?

WHAT CAN YOU DO TO OFFER EMOTIONAL SUPPORT?

❑ *Be with* the dying resident and their family. Spend extra time, hold hands, and talk only when and if they want to talk.

❑ *Reflect* on your own emotional and spiritual response to residents' situations and to dying generally. Manage your own reactions and keep your responses centered on what most helps the residents.

❑ *Listen* with full attention and be sympathetic. Recognize that residents may be suffering emotionally, and that they may become more challenging to care for during this time. Don't take their anger or difficult behaviors personally.

❑ *Allow them choices* in daily routines and care.

❐ *Accept them* for who they are at this time in life. Tell them that you care for them and that you understand this is a hard time.

❐ *Help residents enjoy life,* as many of them prefer to be "living while dying" and find pleasure in ordinary activities and relationships.

❐ *Support special relationships* between residents and staff members by assigning staff caregivers to work with the same residents on a regular basis.

WHAT CAN YOU DO TO OFFER SPIRITUAL SUPPORT?

❐ Listen for spiritual language and concerns, such as referring to God or an afterlife. Don't expect to have easy answers.

❐ Listen with respect and allow questions and anger without offering judgment or solutions.

- Saying "I know this is hard for you" can be comforting

- To hard questions, you may relate the issue back to the resident, such as asking "What do you think?" or "What feels right to you?"

❐ Offer, if you and the resident feel comfortable:

- religious music or hymns

- scripture or devotional reading

- prayer

- sitting together in quietness

- God's forgiveness

❐ Offer to contact a resident's preferred clergy member or a chaplain from hospice.

❐ Encourage the resident and family to reminisce about meaningful events, accomplishments, or relationships in their lives.

❐ Assure residents that they will not be abandoned or forgotten, that they will be cared for well, and that they will be missed when they are gone.

ISSUES TO CONSIDER WHEN HELPING RESIDENTS WITH THEIR EMOTIONAL AND SPIRITUAL NEEDS

❑ Is the resident physically comfortable?

- an uncomfortable resident is less able to cope

- relieve physical discomfort and pain first

❑ Is the resident aware she is dying?

- ask her if she wants to talk about what is happening to her and what to expect in the future—"It must be hard to be so sick. Do you have any concerns about what is going to happen to you?"

- be sensitive to her willingness to talk about her own death—"I care about you and am here if you want to talk about anything."

- include family and other caregivers in discussions

❑ What is the resident's cultural and religious background?

- "Are you a religious or spiritual person? Do you have any beliefs that help you through difficult times?"

❑ What is the resident's emotional and spiritual state?

- "If your time to die should come soon, do you feel ready?"

- "Have you experienced the death of a loved one, and what was that like?"

❑ What are the resident's spiritual resources and inner strengths?

- "How have you coped with hardship in your life?"

- "What has given your life meaning?"

- "Who has helped you or given you strength? Is there anyone—special friends, clergy—who I could ask to come and see you during this difficult time?"

❑ Who are the resident's social support: family, friends, staff, other residents?

- Ask if the resident and family want to be together at the time of death—if so, create a plan to ensure that the family will be called when death is near

- ■ Don't be afraid to let staff or other residents know when a resident is dying—this allows them to say good-bye in whatever way is comfortable for them and the resident

- ■ Allow staff extra time to stay with a dying resident

- ■ Create a private place where family, friends, and other residents can visit

❒ Use the ministry of your time and presence for residents unable to talk about emotional and spiritual needs

- ■ Residents with severe dementia cannot talk about spiritual concerns but may still respond to music or prayer—ask their family what they think the resident would prefer if she or he could talk

- ■ Residents who don't want to talk in religious terms still have emotional needs you can address

- ■ Residents who are angry or in denial are defending themselves from emotional pain—respect where they are in the process of dying, and know that they may not be ready for a frank discussion of their disease or death

- ■ Remember to distinguish between your beliefs and the beliefs and needs of the resident

- ■ Never tell a resident how they should feel or act

❒ Recognize that, for you as a caregiver, it is a special privilege but also a continuing challenge to work with dying people. See the *Participants' Handouts* for this session for a universal prayer that may be helpful to caregivers as they work with residents in emotional and spiritual distress.

THINGS YOU SHOULD RECOGNIZE
AS YOU WORK WITH DYING RESIDENTS

❒ Each death is unique—think of what is individual about this resident's experience.

❒ Ensure physical comfort first.

❒ Acknowledge the emotional and spiritual intensity of dying

- ■ for the resident, this is the final challenge in life

■   for people who love them, this is a very difficult time of loss

❑   Excellent emotional and spiritual care creates a good memory and allows healing for family and staff caregivers.

DISCUSSION: Throughout your career, what are some ways that you have helped dying residents with their emotional and spiritual needs?

Information for Licensed Nursing Staff and Prescribers

Note to Facilitator: The following section (on medications for treating delirium, agitation, and depression) is useful primarily to physicians, nurse practitioners, physician assistants, and licensed nursing staff. Adjust the amount of time you spend on this topic depending on your particular audience.

RECOGNIZING AND TREATING DELIRIUM AND NONSPECIFIC AGITATION

Delirium is an acute or subacute change in mental functioning that is characterized by altered alertness and a fluctuating course. Delirious residents may be increasingly drowsy and spend more time asleep. Alternatively, they may experience an agitated delirium in which they become increasingly alert, physically restless, and have psychotic symptoms such as hallucinations, paranoid ideation, or delusions, for example, thinking an aide is going to take them home. Residents with an agitated delirium may also express strong emotions such as anger, sadness, or anxiety.

Delirium is caused by an underlying organic illness or medication side effect. It occurs more often in residents with dementia than in those who do not have dementia.

When a resident has an acute or subacute change in mental functioning, first test for common causes of delirium:

❑   dehydration, electrolyte imbalance, blood sugars too high or too low

❏   low oxygen saturation, declining kidney function with rising serum creatinine

❏   infections, usually urinary or respiratory; heart attack; or low body temperature

❏   medication effects

❏   alcohol or drug withdrawal

❏   thyroid disease, B12 deficiency

❏   central nervous system causes such as stroke or subdural hematoma (although uncommon causes of delirium)

Treatment of the underlying *cause* is the primary treatment for delirium. Antipsychotic medications may provide symptomatic relief in agitated delirium. Benzodiazepines, such as lorazepam, are usually not effective; they more often worsen delirium. Consider one of the following:

❏   haloperidol 0.5–2.0 mg PO q 6 hours

❏   risperidone 0.5–2.0 mg PO q 6 hours

❏   quetiapine 25–50 mg PO q 12 hours

Nonspecific agitation or anxiety may occur in residents who have underlying dementia. When these symptoms occur in the absence of true delirium or psychotic symptoms, nonpharmacologic interventions are the most effective. In some cases, small doses of benzodiazepines or antipsychotic medications may be helpful if response is monitored carefully.

RECOGNIZING AND TREATING DEPRESSION

Residents who are aware of their progressive illness and functional decline may become depressed.

❏   15% of nursing home residents experience major depression

❏   others may experience constant unhappiness or depressive symptoms without all the symptoms and signs of a major depression

❏   depression among elderly people may be triggered by physical illness, role loss, nursing home placement, or loss of a loved one

❑ elderly individuals who are depressed often describe their mood as anxious or "nervous" rather than sad

Depression is present when a resident has a depressed mood *or* loss of interest and pleasure *and* four of the following symptoms or signs:

❑ weight change

❑ sleep disorder

❑ psychomotor agitation or slowed response

❑ fatigue or loss of energy

❑ feelings of worthlessness or guilt

❑ difficulty concentrating

❑ suicidal thoughts

Antidepressant medication may relieve psychological suffering associated with major depression, even when weight loss and fatigue persist because of a resident's underlying terminal illness. These medications may also provide symptomatic relief for depressive or anxiety symptoms less severe than major depression, when they are taken regularly and their doses are individualized for effective results. Examples of medications to consider are:

❑ Selective Serotonin Reuptake Inhibitors

■ sertraline (Zoloft) 25–150 mg/d

■ paroxetine (Paxil) 10–60 mg/d

❑ Other Antidepressants

■ bupropion (Wellbutrin) 150–300 mg/d *(may be stimulating)*

■ venlafaxine (Effexor) 75–150 mg/d

■ mirtazepine (Remeron) 15–45 mg/d *(can be sedating)*

❑ Psychostimulants

■ methylphenidate (Ritalin) 2.5–10 mg BID

❑ Tricyclic Antidepressants *(these may cause confusion and anticholinergic side effects, such as dry mouth and constipation)*

■ nortriptyline (Pamelor) 10–100 mg/d

- desipramine (Norpramin) 10–150 mg/d

- trazodone (Deseryl) 25–300 mg/hs *(sometimes helpful and safe for sleep)*

Instructions to Facilitator: After going through the material above, move on to the case-based example. Have someone in the group read the example and issues aloud, then pause for discussion. Conclude the session by reading through and discussing the action plan and then distributing the homework.

An Example for Group Discussion and Planning

Case-Based Example: Ms. Barclay

Ms. Barclay, a 95-year-old woman, was "forced" to come to the nursing facility several months ago because of pneumonia, chronic pain for osteoarthritis, alcohol abuse, and falls. She has chronic depression with mild dementia. She also has chronic constipation and bowel incontinence. She is fiercely independent and refuses help with toileting and personal care. She feels angry that her right to live independently has been violated. She refuses to accept psychiatric consultation and believes that everyone else residing in the facility has dementia. Her intake is poor, and she remains in her room, refusing to interact with staff or other residents. Her family members are supportive but feel their interactions with her are tense and not always helpful.

The resident complains of pain under her right arm, and her nurse felt a mass in this area. Her physician ordered a mammogram and breast biopsy, which shows breast cancer with spread to the lymph nodes. The resident has not yet been told of this diagnosis.

Her current medications are nortripyline 10 mg QHS, Vicodin 2 tablets q 6 hours, Percocet q 4 hours PRN, sorbitol, Metamucil, Colace and Ducolax.

Issues to Consider

❐ *This resident is angry, depressed, refusing care, and in denial.*

❐ *Bowel incontinence and her unwillingness to accept help create problems for her skin, sanitation, and odor.*

❐ *Pain control is inadequate.*

❐ *Ms. Barclay needs help with social isolation and poor quality of life.*

❐ *She has so many needs it is hard to know how to begin. What is the first, best step that you as a team can take to improve care for this suffering resident?*

STOP: Discuss the above case before going on to the action plan. How do you recommend working with Ms. Barclay?

An Action Plan for Ms. Barclay

First Steps:

❐ Establish a therapeutic relationship

  ■ Acknowledge that living in the nursing home is not how or where she wants to live, and that you know it is very hard for her

  ■ Listen to what is most important to her, and promise to work with her to meet her needs

❐ Treat her pain

  ■ Stop Vicodin and Percocet and begin a dose-equivalent, long-acting opioid (e.g., MS Contin) plus a short-acting opioid to be increased as needed (e.g., morphine)

Next Steps:

❐ A nurse who has a trusting relationship with Ms. Barclay asks her what she thinks is causing the pain under her arm, and finds out how much she wants to know about her disease.

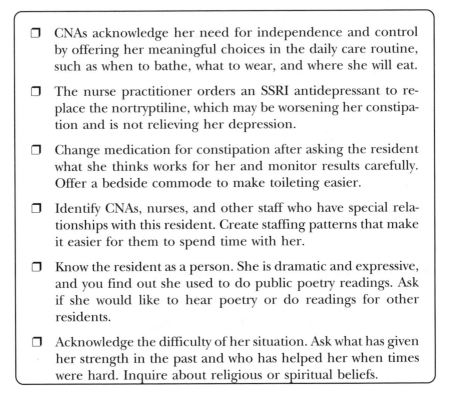

❏ CNAs acknowledge her need for independence and control by offering her meaningful choices in the daily care routine, such as when to bathe, what to wear, and where she will eat.

❏ The nurse practitioner orders an SSRI antidepressant to replace the nortryptiline, which may be worsening her constipation and is not relieving her depression.

❏ Change medication for constipation after asking the resident what she thinks works for her and monitor results carefully. Offer a bedside commode to make toileting easier.

❏ Identify CNAs, nurses, and other staff who have special relationships with this resident. Create staffing patterns that make it easier for them to spend time with her.

❏ Know the resident as a person. She is dramatic and expressive, and you find out she used to do public poetry readings. Ask if she would like to hear poetry or do readings for other residents.

❏ Acknowledge the difficulty of her situation. Ask what has given her strength in the past and who has helped her when times were hard. Inquire about religious or spiritual beliefs.

DISCUSSION: Finish the session with further discussion about the importance of addressing spiritual and emotional needs when providing end-of-life care.

ANNOTATED BIBLIOGRAPHY

Note to Facilitator: Before you present this session, if you would like to learn more about emotional and spiritual care of nursing home residents, we suggest the following materials.

Callahan, M., & Kelley, P. (1992). *Final Gifts: Understanding the Special Awareness, Needs, and Communications of the Dying.* New York: Poseidon Press.
This interesting and easy-to-read book is written by two long-time hospice nurses. They use case examples to discuss helpful methods of working with dying individuals and their families, placing a special emphasis on the psychological, emotional, and spiritual needs of this population.

Conrad, N. L. (1985). Spiritual support for the dying. *Nursing Clinics of North America*, *20*, 415–426.

This author asserts that the spiritual needs of the dying generally fall into four categories: a search for meaning, a sense of forgiveness, hope, and love. She argues that nurses are in a good position to help their patients address these needs, because "nurses are easily accepted into a client's intimate sphere during the course of their physical care, and intimacy in the spiritual dimension can follow naturally for nurses who are alert to this possibility." The article offers examples of ways in which nursing staff can help address patients' spiritual needs, such as asking the patient if they can pray together, encouraging life review, reading to the patient, or leading the patient through guided mediation or imagery.

Hicks, T. J., Jr. (1999). Spirituality and the elderly: Nursing implications with nursing home residents. *Geriatric Nursing, 20*, 144–146.

This article lists three ways in which nurses can assist nursing home residents in their spiritual journeys: by silent witnessing, by serving as a liaison for residents' needs, and through active listening. The author suggests how nursing home staff can best assess residents' spiritual needs and encourages attention to spiritual needs as a routine part of care planning.

Lo, B., Ruston, D., Kates, L. W., Arnold, R. M., Cohen, C. B., Faber-Langendoen, K., et al. (2002). Discussing religious and spiritual issues at the end of life. *JAMA, 287*, 749–754.

These authors, from the *Working Group on Religious and Spiritual Issues at the End of Life*, offer concrete suggestions as to how physicians and other health care professionals might respond when patients or their families raise spiritual or religious concerns. They give examples of "phrases to help elicit the patient's concerns" and discuss some of the "pitfalls" that health care providers can encounter when discussing spiritual and religious issues with their patients, as well as advising how best to avoid these mistakes.

8

Caring for the Caregiver: Taking Care of Yourself Emotionally

---

Note to Facilitator: The main objective of this session is to help caregivers reflect on their feelings about death and about experiences as a caregiver. The exercises encourage staff to understand their own experiences with death and to learn how to work better as a team. You should allow time for them to share their stories, feelings, and concerns throughout the session. *Time Estimate: 60 minutes.*

OVERVIEW

Many caregivers and health professionals believe they are expected to be "strong" in the face of pain, suffering, and death and to avoid showing feelings in the workplace. We know, however, that caring for dying residents is stressful under the best of circumstances. When someone you care for dies, you might feel like never getting attached again, just to protect yourself. However, in this special work you do with dying residents and their families, there are other ways to cope with sadness and to find rewards in your work. After a resident dies, staff members need to remember the resident, to share feelings with others, to grieve, and to get support from others. This session will discuss strategies that nursing home staff can use to cope with the stresses they encounter in their difficult but extremely important line of work.

As you move through this session, remember:

❐   that caring for yourself is essential for survival in this work

❐   that caring for yourself will enable you to give good care to your residents

❐   to listen during this session for new ideas about how to care for yourself

The goal of this session is to learn how we can take care of ourselves and our team, in order to be strong enough to continue caring for dying residents.

> **Instructions to Facilitator:** Read the following question and statements to encourage the group to talk about stressful experiences they have had when caring for dying residents. Plan to spend about 10 minutes sharing stories of challenges and frustrations. Tell the participants that time for this discussion is short, so they should try to summarize their stories.

CARING FOR DYING NURSING HOME RESIDENTS CAN BE VERY STRESSFUL

We all know that caring for a resident who is dying can be very difficult. Do any of these situations remind you of a stressful time in your own work?

❐   You came to work and found out that a resident you cared for had died

❐   You were asked to bathe and turn a resident who seemed to be in terrible pain

❐   One of your coworkers is unable to come to work; as a result, you have four extra residents assigned to you, one of whom is dying

❐   One of your dying residents has a family who is fighting over whether or not the resident should be sent to the hospital

❐   It just seems to you that every week a resident you care about has died

❐ You feel like crying when one of your residents has just died, but your supervisor tells you that there is no time for this, you have a new admission to go see

STOP: Spend time discussing some of the stresses you encounter in working with dying nursing home residents.

Instructions to Facilitator: Read the following question and statements, then ask the group to spend about 10 minutes discussing ways they find their work to be rewarding and satisfying.

CARING FOR DYING NURSING HOME RESIDENTS CAN BE DEEPLY REWARDING

Caring for a resident who is dying can be one of the most valuable and rewarding aspects of this difficult work. Do any of these situations remind you of a special time in your own work?

❐ You were with one of your favorite residents when she died, and she looked clean, comfortable, and peaceful

❐ You noticed that a new aide was frightened when she was asked to clean the body of a resident who had died, and you showed her how to do it

❐ The charge nurse complimented you because you reported a resident being in pain and then followed up with a report of how he responded to pain medication

❐ Your work has helped you to appreciate the value of life every day and has helped your own family face death

❐ Because you know a dying resident is religious and loves gospel music, you invite a pastor to visit her and you set up taped gospel music in her room

STOP: Spend time discussing some of the rewards and good experiences you have had in your work with the dying.

Instructions to Facilitator: Read through the remainder of the comments quickly, to encourage people to think about how they care for themselves and each other. The reading should be brief, about 5 minutes. Then open discussion so that the group can respond to the material. Finish the session by passing out the homework.

WHAT KNOWLEDGE AND SKILLS DO YOU NEED TO KEEP WORKING WITH DYING RESIDENTS?

You need to know that:

❐ *Everyone who works with dying residents has to cope with the feelings they have about death.* Recognize that a dying resident may bring up feelings of sadness from previous deaths or remind you of your own death in the future.

❐ *Grieving for someone who died is human and natural.* If you are sad after a resident dies, it is a sign that you cared for that person. Your attachment to her probably allowed you to provide better care while she was alive.

❐ *Sadness and grief are not the only emotions after death; be honest with yourself about what you really feel.* You may not grieve for a resident if you weren't attached to him. You may feel relief that his suffering is over, celebration of a life well-lived, or satisfaction with the care you gave and the love his family showed.

You will feel better if you:

❐ *Call on your own sources of strength when coping with loss and grief.* You might find comfort remembering the person who died, praying, or thinking about what gives you spiritual strength in the face of death. You can reflect on what you were able to give this person as she was preparing to die, and forgive yourself for things you didn't do. You may acknowledge that each death is a learning experience and ask yourself how you could do things differently when your next resident dies.

❐ *Find support from others.* Share how you feel about losing this particular resident. Tell stories about the resident with family, staff, and other residents who also may feel grief or other reactions to the loss. If possible, find time to do this soon after the death.

❐ *Think about how hardships have made you a stronger person.* Some ways to do this are to:

- look at a hard situation as a challenge or a problem you can solve

- accept that there are some problems you can't solve, but feel good about the ways you can help

❐ *Feel proud of your commitment to this valuable work.*

❐ *Look for continuing education opportunities in end-of-life care.* Learning new skills makes you feel more capable and comfortable as a caregiver for dying residents.

HOW CAN YOU WORK BETTER AS A TEAM OF CAREGIVERS?

❐ Ask for help from others when you find caring for a resident or family member difficult.

❐ When a resident is dying, ask what you can do to help another team member.

❐ Find someone you trust and share worries, secrets, or mistakes with that person.

❐ Mentor and teach new employees so they begin to feel comfortable with this work.

❐ Communicate!

- Ask the nurse or doctor what is happening to a resident so you feel more informed

- Tell other team members when you find something that works to keep a dying resident comfortable, and ask that this idea be added to the care plan

- Compliment coworkers who are doing a good job

- Stop and offer support to a coworker who is having a difficult time emotionally

HOW CAN YOU SAY GOOD-BYE?

Saying good-bye is something we all need to do when someone is dying, although we may not necessarily use the word "goodbye." Here are some ideas for making this part of the good care you give dying residents and each other:

❐ Let your dying resident know how special she is to you and that you have enjoyed caring for her.

❐ When it feels right, tell your dying resident good-bye and that you will miss him when he is gone.

❐ When a resident dies, let other residents and staff know what has happened. Give other residents time to respond, and say something supportive to them, like "I know you will miss her."

❐ Take time with coworkers to tell stories and share feelings. You may do this informally or ask the facility social worker or hospice chaplain to facilitate this.

❐ Memorials are an important way for the nursing home to help everyone

   ▪ Have a memorial service in the facility for staff, other residents, and family

   ▪ Set up a memory book for people to write memories under a picture of the resident. This can be copied for the staff to keep in the facility, and the original can be given as a gift to the family

   ▪ Ask for time off to attend the funeral or memorial service

DISCUSSION: What do we need to do for ourselves and our team to make us all stronger caregivers for dying residents?

ANNOTATED BIBLIOGRAPHY

Note to Facilitator: Before you present this session, if you would like to learn more about helping nursing home staff cope with death on the job, we suggest the following articles.

Eakes, G. G. (1990). Grief resolution in hospice nurses: An exploration of effective methods. *Nursing and Health Care, 11,* 242–248.

The author of this article spoke with hospice nurses about how they cope with the cumulative effect of dealing with dying patients on an ongoing basis. Some of the tips the nurses offered included working with patients and families to develop "comfort" rather than "cure" goals, sharing their feelings of grief and pain honestly with families and with one another, seeking closure in relationships with families (for example, by attending funeral services), and having a positive attitude towards the elderly.

Genevay, B. (Fall 1994). Roses and onions: The fruits of helping old and dying people. *Generations, 18,* 13–15.

This article outlines some of the challenges and difficulties, but also the benefits, of being a front-line worker in a nursing home setting. The "roses," or rewards, of caring for the dying elderly include the opportunity for growth as one confronts aging, disability, and dying; the ability to find new perspectives on issues of power and control; and the joy that can result from achieving and exchanging intimacy with older people.

Herrle, S. M. (September 1987). Helping staff cope with grief. *Nursing Management, 18,* 33–34.

The author of this article, a nurse in a hospital oncology unit, describes her strategy for organizing workplace-based grief sessions for staff to help them cope with deaths they witness on their jobs.

Marino, P. A. (1998). The effects of cumulative grief in the nurse. *Journal of Intravenous Nursing, 21,* 101–104.

Marino describes organizational and psychosocial stressors affecting those who work closely with the dying. She then describes strategies that both institutions and individuals can use to minimize the effects of stress and cumulative grief. Coping strategies include worksite education and training, opportunities for staff support and team-building, flexibility in the workplace, and balance in our lives.

References

Acello, B. (April 2001). Focus on pain: The nurse assistant's role in pain management. *Journal of Nurse Assistants,* 18–32.

Ackerman, T. F. (1997). Forsaking the spirit for the letter of the law: Advance directives in nursing homes. *Journal of the American Geriatrics Society, 45,* 114–116.

Ahronheim, J. C. (1996). Nutrition and hydration in the terminal patient. *Clinics in Geriatric Medicine, 12,* 379–391.

American Geriatrics Society Panel on Chronic Pain in Older Persons (1998). The management of chronic pain in older persons. *Journal of the American Geriatrics Society, 46,* 635–651.

Ausdenmoore, M. M. (April 1998). A touching moment: Using an age-old healing technique to ease a client's death. *Nursing, 28,* 32hh6.

Baer, W. M., & Hanson, L. C. (2000). Families perceptions of the added value of hospice in the nursing home. *Journal of the American Geriatrics Society, 48,* 879–882.

Bascom, P. B., & Tolle, S. W. (1995). Care of the family when the patient is dying, in *Caring for patients at the end of life* [Special Issue]. *Western Journal of Medicine, 163,* 292–296.

Beaudoin, S. J. (Aug. 1990). Caring and surviving. *Canadian Nurse, 86,* 19–20.

Bernabei, R., Gambassi, G., Lapane, K., Landi, F., Gatsonis, C., Dunlop, R., et al. (1998). Management of pain in elderly patients with cancer. *Journal of the American Medical Association, 279,* 1877–1882.

Block, S. D. (2001). Psychological considerations, growth, and transcendence at the end of life: The art of the possible. *Journal of the American Medical Association, 285,* 2898–2905.

Block, S. D. (2000). Assessing and managing depression in the terminally ill patient. *Annals of Internal Medicine, 132,* 209–218.

Bottrell, M. M., O'Sullivan, J. E., Robbins, M. A., Mitty, E. L., & Mezey, M. D. (2001). Transferring dying nursing home residents to the hospital: DON perspectives on the nurse's role in transfer decisions. *Geriatric Nursing, 22,* 313–317.

Bradley, E., Walker, L., Blechner, B., & Wetle, T. (1997). Assessing capacity to participate in discussions of advance directives in nursing homes: Findings from a study of the patient self determination act. *Journal of the American Geriatrics Society, 45,* 79–83.

British Medical Journal Editorial Board (2000). A good death. *British Medical Journal, 320,* 129–130.

Buckingham, R. W. (Spring 1983). Hospice in a long-term care facility: An innovative pattern of care. *Journal of Long-Term Care Administration, 11,* 10–14.

Byock, I. R. (1995). Patient refusal of nutrition and hydration: Walking the ever-finer line. *American Journal of Hospice & Palliative Care, 12,* 8–13.

Callahan, M., & Kelley, P. (1992). *Final Gifts: Understanding the Special Awareness, Needs, and Communications of the Dying.* New York: Poseidon Press.

Chekryn, J. (May/June 1985). Support for the family of the dying patient. *Home Healthcare Nurse, 3,* 18–24.

Churchill, L., Doron, M., Rothman, E., & Yarger, L. (2000). Video: *Those Who Stay Behind: When a Family Member is Dying.* Boston: Fanlight Productions.

Conrad, N. L. (1985). Spiritual support for the dying. *Nursing Clinics of North America, 20,* 415–426.

Coolican, M. B., Stark, J., Doka, K. J., & Corr, C. A. (November/December 1994). Education about death, dying, and bereavement in nursing programs. *Nurse Educator, 19,* 35–40.

Corr, C. A., & Doka, K. J. (1994). Current models of death, dying, and bereavement. *Critical Care Nursing Clinics of North America, 6,* 545–552.

Crawley, L., Payne, R., Bolden, J., Payne, T., Washington, P., Williams, S. (2000). Palliative and end-of-life care in the African-American community. *Journal of the American Medical Association, 284,* 2518–2521.

Crawley, L. M., Marshall, P. A., Lo, B., & Koenig, B. A. (2002). Strategies for culturally effective end-of-life care. *Annals of Internal Medicine, 136,* 673–679.

Daly, B. J. (Sept. 2000). Special challenges of withholding artificial nutrition and hydration. *Journal of Gerontological Nursing, 26,* 25–31.

Degner, L. F., Gow, C. M., & Thompson, L. A. (1991). Critical nursing behaviors in care for the dying. *Cancer Nursing, 14,* 246–253.

Dorner, B., Gallagher-Allred, C., Deering, C. P., & Posthauer M. E. (1997). The 'to feed or not to feed' dilemma. *Journal of the American Dietetic Association, 97*(Suppl 2), S172–S176.

Doyle, D. (1992). Have we looked beyond the physical and psychosocial? *Journal of Pain and Symptom Management, 7,* 302–311.

Dunn, H. (2001). *Hard Choices for Loving People.* Herndon, VA: ANA Publishing.

Eakes, G. G. (1990). Grief resolution in hospice nurses: An exploration of effective methods. *Nursing and Health Care, 11,* 242–248.

Engle, V. F. (1998). Care of the living, care of the dying: Reconceptualizing nursing home care. *Journal of the American Geriatrics Society, 46,* 1172–1174.

Engle, V. F., Fox-Hill, E., & Graney, M. J. (1998). The experience of living-dying in a nursing home: Self-reports of black and white older adults. *Journal of the American Geriatrics Society, 46,* 1091–1096.

Ersek, M., Kraybill, B. M., & Hansberry, J. (October 2000). Assessing the educational needs and concerns of nursing staff regarding end-of-life care. *Journal of Gerontological Nursing, 26,* 16–26.

Ersek, M., Kraybill, B. M., & Hansberry, J. (1999). Investigating the educational needs of licensed nursing staff and certified nursing assistants in nursing homes regarding end-of-life care. *American Journal of Hospice & Palliative Care, 16,* 573–582.

Evans, M. A., Esbenson, M., & Jaffe, C. (December 1981). Expect the unexpected when you care for a dying patient. *Nursing, 11,* 55–56.

Feinsod, F. M., Prochoda, K. P., Anneberg, A. L., & Solomon, W. (2000). The medical director's role in pain management for residents in long-term care facilities. *Annals of Long-Term Care, 8,* 43–48.

Feldt, K. S., Warne, M. A., & Ryden, M. B. (November 1998). Examining pain in aggressive cognitively impaired older adults. *Journal of Gerontological Nursing, 24,* 14–22.

Ferrell, B. A. (1995). Pain evaluation and management in the nursing home. *Annals of Internal Medicine, 123,* 681–687.

Ferrell, B. A., Ferrell, B. R., & Rivera, L. (1995). Pain in cognitively impaired nursing home patients. *Journal of Pain and Symptom Management, 10,* 591–598.

Finucane, T. E., Christmas, C., & Travis, K. (1999). Tube feeding in patients with advanced dementia: A review of the evidence. *Journal of the American Medical Association, 282,* 1365–1370.

Fischer, G. S., Arnold, R. M., & Tulsky, J. A. (2000). Talking to the older adult about advance directives. *Clinics in Geriatric Medicine, 16,* 239–254.

Flacker, J. M., & Kiely, D. K. (1998). A practical approach to identifying mortality-related factors in established long-term care residents. *Journal of the American Geriatrics Society, 46,* 1012–1015.

Fox, P. L., Raina, P., & Jadad, A. R. (1999). Prevalence and treatment of pain in older adults in nursing homes and other long-term care institutions: A systematic review. *Canadian Medical Association Journal, 160,* 329–333.

Froggatt, K., Hasnip, J., & Smith, P. (April 2000). The challenges of end of life care. *Elderly Care, 12,* 11–13.

Genevay, B. (Fall 1994). Roses and onions: The fruits of helping old and dying people. *Generations, 18,* 13–15.

Gross, D. (September/October 1999). Dealing with death in the nursing home. *Balance, 3,* 12–13.

Herrle, S. M. (September 1987). Helping staff cope with grief. *Nursing Management, 18,* 33–34.

Hicks, T. J., Jr. (1999). Spirituality and the elderly: Nursing implications with nursing home residents. *Geriatric Nursing, 20,* 144–146.

Jackonen, S. (July-September 1997). Dehydration and hydration in the terminally ill: Care considerations. *Nursing Forum, 32,* 5–13.

Hallenbeck, J., Goldstein, M. K., & Mebane, E. W. (1996). Cultural considerations of death and dying in the United States. *Clinics in Geriatric Medicine, 12,* 393–406.

Hanson, L. C., & Henderson, M. (2000). Care of the dying in long-term care settings. *Clinics in Geriatric Medicine, 16,* 225–237.

Hanson, L. C., Henderson, M., & Menon, M. (2002). As individual as death itself: A focus group study of terminal care in nursing homes. *Journal of Palliative Medicine, 5,* 117–125.

Hayley, D. C., Cassel, C. K., Snyder, L., & Rudberg, M. A. (1996). Ethical and legal issues in nursing home care. *Archives of Internal Medicine, 156,* 249–256.

Hicks, T. J. (1999). Spirituality and the elderly: Nursing implications with nursing home residents. *Geriatric Nursing, 20,* 144–146.

Holstein, M. (1997). Reflections on death and dying. *Academic Medicine, 72,* 848–855.

Horgas, A. L., & Dunn, K. (March 2001). Pain in nursing home residents: Comparison of residents' self-report and nursing assistants' perceptions. *Journal of Gerontological Nursing, 27,* 44–53.

Horgas, A. L., & Tsai, P. F. (1998). Analgesic drug prescription and use in cognitively impaired nursing home residents. *Nursing Research, 47,* 235–242.

Hurley, A. C., Volicer, B. J., Hanrahan, P. A., Houde, S., & Volicer, L. (1992). Assessment of discomfort in advanced alzheimer patients. *Research in Nursing and Health, 15,* 369–377.

Kagawa-Singer, M., & Blackhall, L. J. (2001). Negotiating cross-cultural issues at the end of life. *Journal of the American Medical Association, 286,* 2993–3001.

Kamel, H. K., Phlavan, M., Malekgoudarzi, B., Gogel, P., & Morley, J. E. (2001). Utilizing pain assessment scales increased the frequency of diagnosing pain among elderly nursing home residents. *Journal of Pain and Symptom Management, 21,* 450–455.

Katsma, D. L., & Souza, C. H. (September 2000). Elderly pain assessment and pain management knowledge of long-term care nurses. *Pain Management Nursing, 1,* 88–95.

Keay, T. J., Alexander, C., McNally, K., Crusse, B., Eger, R. E., Hawtin, C., et al. (2000). Adult education program in palliative care for nursing facility physicians: Design and pilot test. *Journal of Palliative Medicine, 3,* 457–463.

Keay, T. J., Fredman, L., Taler, G. A., Datta, S., & Levenson, S. A. (1994). Indicators of quality medical care for the terminally ill in nursing homes. *Journal of the American Geriatrics Society, 42,* 853–860.

Keay, T. J., & Schonwetter, R. S. (1998). Hospice care in the nursing home. *American Family Physician, 57,* 491–494.

Keay, T. J., Taler, G. A., Fredman, L., & Levenson, S. A. (1997). Assessing medical care of dying residents in nursing homes. *American Journal of Medical Quality, 12,* 151–156.

Kinzel, T. (March/April 1992). Treat pain aggressively to improve resident comfort. *Nursing Homes, 41,* 27–29.

Koenig, H. G., Weiner, D. K., Peterson, B. L., Meador, K. G., & Keefe, F. J. (1997). Religious coping in the nursing home: A biopsychosocial model. *International Journal of Psychiatry in Medicine, 27,* 365–376.

Kovach, C. R., Weissman, D. E., Griffie, J., Matson, S., & Muchka, S. (1999). Assessment and treatment of discomfort for people with late-stage dementia. *Journal of Pain and Symptom Management, 18,* 412–419.

Kovach, C. R., Noonan, P. E., Griffie, J., Muchka, S., & Weissman, D. E. (March 2002). The assessment of discomfort in dementia protocol. *Pain Management Nursing, 3,* 16–27.

Krigger, K. W., McNeely, J. D., & Lippmann, S. B. (1997). Death, dying, and grief: Helping patients and their families through the process. *Postgraduate Medicine, 101,* 263–270.

Krohn, B. (1998). When death is near: Helping families cope. *Geriatric Nursing, 19,* 276–278.

Kubler-Ross, E. (Nov. 1991). Letter to a nurse about death and dying. *Nursing, 21,* 78–80.

Kubler-Ross, E. (1969). *On Death and Dying.* New York: Macmillan.

Lahn, M., Friedman, B., Bijur, P., Haughey, M., & Gallagher, E. J. (2001). Advance directives in skilled nursing facility residents transferred to emergency departments. *Academic Emergency Medicine, 8,* 1158–1162.

Lander, M., Wilson, K., & Chochinov, H. M. (2000). Depression and the dying older patient. *Clinics in Geriatric Medicine, 16,* 335–356.

Lannie, V. J. (May 1978). The joy of caring for the dying. *Supervisor Nurse, 9,* 66–72.

Lethem, W. (November 3, 1999). Nursing home nurses deliver palliative care. *Nursing Times, 95,* 54–55.

Lo, B., et al. (2002). Discussing religious and spiritual issues at the end of life. *Journal of the American Medical Association, 287,* 749–754.

LoCicero, J. P. (May 1997). Grief, long-term care, and hospice: A partnership to enhance the quality of life of dying patients. *Home Health Care Management Practice, 9,* 31–35.

Long, M. C. (1996). Death and dying and recognizing approaching death. *Clinics in Geriatric Medicine, 12,* 359–367.

Luchins, D. J., & Hanrahan, P. (1993). What is appropriate health care for end-stage dementia? *Journal of the American Geriatrics Society, 41,* 25–30.

Luchins, D. J., Hanrahan, P., & Murphy, K. (1997). Criteria for enrolling dementia patients in hospice. *Journal of the American Geriatrics Society, 45,* 1054–1059.

Lynn, J. (2001). Serving patients who may die soon and their families: The role of hospice and other services. *Journal of the American Medical Association, 285,* 925–932.

McCaffery, M. (August 1998). Pain relief for the dying. *Nursing, 28,* 6.

McCaffery, M., & Ferrell, B. R. (1997). Nurses' knowledge of pain assessment and management: How much progress have we made? *Journal of Pain and Symptom Management, 14,* 175–188.

McMann, R. M., Hall, W. J., & Groth-Juncker, A. (1994). Comfort care for terminally ill patients: The appropriate use of nutrition and hydration. *Journal of the American Medical Association, 272,* 1263–1266.

Marino, P. A. (1998). The effects of cumulative grief in the nurse. *Journal of Intravenous Nursing, 21,* 101–104.

Martin, D. K., Emanuel, L. L., & Singer, P. A. (2000). Planning for the end of life. *Lancet, 356,* 1672–1676.

Meares, C. J. (1997). Primary caregiver perceptions of intake cessation in patients who are terminally ill. *Oncology Nursing Forum, 24,* 1751–1757.

Mears, D. (July 1990). Enhancing family coping skills. *Nursing Homes, 39,* 32–33.

Medical College of Wisconsin (2000). *Nursing Staff Education Resource Manual: Pain Management 101.* Milwaukee: Author.

Medical College of Wisconsin (1998). *Improving Pain Management in Long Term Care Settings: A Resource Guide for Institutional Change.* Milwaukee: Author.

Meier, D. E., Morrison, R. S., & Cassel, C. K. (1997). Improving palliative care. *Annals of Internal Medicine, 127,* 225–230.

Mezey, M. D., & Dubler, N. N. (Eds.) (2001). *Voices of Decision in Nursing Homes: Respecting Residents' Preferences for End-of-Life Care.* New York: United Hospital Fund.

Mezey, M., Dubler, N., Lo, B., Engle, V., & Arno, P. (1996). *Decisions about death in long-term care: Development and dissemination of guidelines to ease the death of residents in nursing homes.* New York: New York University Retirement Research Foundation.

Mezey, M., Mitty, E. L., Bottrell, M. M., Ramsey, G. C., & Fisher, T. (2000). Advance directives: Older adults with dementia. *Clinics in Geriatric Medicine, 16,* 255–268.

Mezey, M., Mitty, E., & Ramsey, G. (March 1997). Assessment of decision-making capacity: Nursing's role. *Journal of Gerontological Nursing, 23,* 28–35.

Miller, K. E., Miller, M. M., & Jolley, M. R. (2001). Challenges in pain management at the end of life. *American Family Physician, 64,* 1227–1234.

Miller, L. L., Nelson, L. L., & Mezey, M. (September 2000). Comfort and pain relief in dementia: Awakening a new beneficence. *Journal of Gerontological Nursing, 26*, 33–40.

Miller, S. C., Gozalo, P., & Mor, V. (2001). Hospice enrollment and hospitalization of dying nursing home patients. *American Journal of Medicine, 111*, 38–44.

Miller, S. L., Kiely, D. K., & Lipsitz, L. A. (1998). Does artificial entral nutrition prolong the survival of institutionalized elders with chewing and swallowing problems? *Journal of Gerontology: Medical Sciences, 53A*, M207–M213.

Mitchell, S. L., Tetroe, J., & O'Connor, A. M. (2001). A decision aid for long-term tube feeding in cognitively impaired older persons. *Journal of the American Geriatrics Society, 49*, 313–316.

Morris, E. (October 1988). A pain of separation. *Nursing Times, 84*, 54–56.

Morrison, R. S., & Morris, J. (July 1995). When there is no cure: Palliative care for the dying patient. *Geriatrics, 50*, 45–53.

Morrison, R. S., & Siu, A. L. (2000). Survival in end-state dementia following acute illness. *Journal of the American Medical Association, 284*, 47–52.

Morrison, R. S., Zayas, L. H., Mulvihill, M., Baskin, S. A., & Meier, D. E. (1998). Barriers to completion of health care proxy forms: A qualitative analysis of ethnic differences. *Journal of Clinical Ethics, 9*, 118–126.

Munley, A., Powers, C. S., & Williamson, J. B. (1982). Humanizing nursing home environments: The relevance of hospice principles. *International Journal of Aging and Human Development, 15*, 263–284.

Palker, N. B., & Nettles-Carlson, B. (February 1995). The prevalence of advance directives: Lessons from a nursing home. *Nurse Practitioner, 20*, 7–8, 13, 17–18.

Parkash, R., & Burge, F. (Winter 1997). The family's perspective on issues of hydration in terminal care. *Journal of Palliative Care, 13*, 23–27.

Pasero, C., & McCaffery, M. (November 2001). The undertreatment of pain. *American Journal of Nursing, 101*, 62–65.

Perkins, H. S., Geppert, C. M. A., Gonzales, A., Cortez, J. D., & Hazuda, H. P. (2002). Cross-cultural similarities and differences in attitudes about advance care planning. *Journal of General Internal Medicine, 17*, 48–57.

Pierce, S. F. (April-June 1999). Improving end-of-life care: Gathering suggestions from family members. *Nursing Forum, 34*, 5–14.

Piles, C. L. (January/February 1990). Providing spiritual care. *Nurse Educator, 15*, 36–41.

Printz, L. A. (1992). Terminal dehydration, a compassionate treatment. *Archives of Internal Medicine, 152*, 697–700.

Puchalski, C. M. (2003). Spirituality and end-of-life care: A time for listening and caring. *Journal of Palliative Medicine, 5*, 289–294.

Reagan, J. E., Tulsky, J. A., & Fox, E. (2002). Advance care planning by proxy for residents of long-term care facilities who lack decision-making capacity. *Journal of the American Geriatrics Society, 50*, 761–767.

Reynolds, K. S., Henderson, M., Schulman, A., & Hanson, L. C. (2002). Needs of the dying in nursing homes. *Journal of Palliative Medicine, 5*, 895–901.

Riesenberg, D. (2000). Hospital care of patients with dementia. *Journal of the American Medical Association, 284*, 87–89.

Roter, D. L., Larson, S., Fischer, G. S., Arnold, R. M., & Tulsky, J. A. (2000). Experts practice what they preach: A descriptive study of best and normative practices in end-of-life discussions. *Archives of Internal Medicine, 160*, 3477–3485.

Sander, R., & Russell, P. (April 2001). Care for dying people in nursing homes. *Nursing Older People, 13,* 21–24.

Scheel, B. J., & Lynn, J. (1988). Care of dying patients. *Clinics in Geriatric Medicine, 4,* 639–654.

Sengstaken, E. A., & King, S. A. (1993). The problems of pain and its detection among geriatric nursing home residents. *Journal of the American Geriatrics Society, 41,* 541–544.

Seskevich, J. (2000). *Guided Relaxation with Touch Therapy* (Video). Durham, NC: Stress Management Education.

Shuster, J. L. (2000). Palliative care for advanced dementia. *Clinics in Geriatric Medicine, 16,* 373–386.

Singer, P. A., Martin, D. K., Lavery, S. V., Thiel, E. C., Kelner, M., & Mendelssohn, D. C. (1998). Reconceptualizing advance care planning from the patient's perspective. *Archives of Internal Medicine, 158,* 879–884.

Singer, P. A., Martin, D. K., & Kelner, M. (1999). Quality end-of-life care: Patients' perspectives. *Journal of the American Medical Association, 281,* 163–168.

Smith, S. A., & Andrews, M. (2000). Artificial nutrition and hydration at the end of life. *MEDSURG Nursing, 9,* 233–244.

Steele, K., Ribbe, M., Ahronheim, J., Hedrick, H., Selwyn, P. A., Forman, W., et al. (1999). Incorporating education on palliative care into the long-term care setting. *Journal of the American Geriatrics Society, 47,* 904–907.

Stein, W. M. (2001). Pain in the nursing home. *Clinics in Geriatric Medicine, 17,* 575–594.

Stein, W. M., & Ferrell, B. A. (1996). Pain in the nursing home. *Clinics in Geriatric Medicine, 12,* 601–613.

Steinhauser, K. E., Clipp, E. C., McNeilly, M., Christakis, N. A., McIntyre, L. M., Tulsky, J. A. (2000). In search of a good death: Observations of patients, families, and providers. *Annals of Internal Medicine, 132,* 825–832.

Teno, J. M., Casey, V. A., Welch, L. C., & Edgman-Levitan, S. (2001). Patient-focused, family-centered, end-of-life medical care: Views of the guidelines and bereaved family members. *Journal of Pain and Symptom Management, 22,* 738–751.

Vachon, M. L. S. (Autumn 1998). Psychosocial needs of patients and families. *Journal of Palliative Care, 14,* 49–56.

Von Gunten, C. F., Ferris, F. D., & Emanuel, L. L. (2000). Ensuring competency in end-of-life care: Communication and relational skills. *Journal of the American Medical Association, 284,* 3051–3057.

Welk, T. A. (November 1998). Beyond pain: A team approach. *American Journal of Nursing, 98,* 16NN–16PP.

Wheeler, S. R. (July 1996). Helping families cope with death and dying. *Nursing, 26,* 25–31.

Whitecar, P. S., Jonas, A. P., & Clasen, M. E. (2000). Managing pain in the dying patient. *American Family Physician, 61,* 755–764.

Wills, A. (December 14, 1988). The final journey. *Nursing Times, 84,* 27–28.

Wilson, S. A., & Daley, B. J. (November 1999). Family perspectives on dying in long-term care settings. *Journal of Gerontological Nursing, 25,* 19–25.

Wilson, S. A., & Daley, B. J. (1998). Attachment/detachment: Forces influencing care of the dying in long-term care. *Journal of Palliative Medicine, 1,* 21–34.

Wilson, S. A., Kovach, C. R., & Stearns, S. A. (1996). Hospice concepts in the care of end-stage dementia. *Geriatric Nursing, 17,* 6–10.

Won, A., Lapane, K., Gambassi, G., Bernabei, R., Mor, V., & Lipsitz, L. A. (1999). Correlates and management of nonmalignant pain in the nursing home. *Journal of the American Geriatrics Society, 47,* 936–942.

Wong, D. L., & Baker, C. M. (2001). Smiling faces as anchor for pain intensity scales. *Pain, 89,* 295–300.

Wong, D. L., & Baker, C. M. (1988). Pain in children: Comparison of assessment scales. *Pediatric Nursing, 14,* 9–17.

Yeh, S. S., Wu, S. Y., Lee, T. P., Olson, J. S., Steins, M. R., Dixon, T., et al. (2000). Improvement in quality-of-life measures and stimulation of weight gain after treatment with megestrol acetate oral suspension in geriatric cachexia: Results of a double-blind, placebo-controlled study. *Journal of the American Geriatrics Society, 48,* 485–492.

Your turn. (July 1998). *Journal of Gerontological Nursing, 24,* 47–52.

Zerwekh, J. V. (March 1997). Do dying patients really need IV fluids? *American Journal of Nursing, 97,* 26–31.

Prognostic Guidelines

Flacker Mortality Score

Using the Flacker Mortality Score and the Resident Assessment Instrument to Identify Residents at High Risk for Dying Within One Year[1]

For each resident, complete the chart below and tabulate a total score:

Resident: _____ Date: _____

Resident Characteristic	Scoring Chart	Score
Functional Ability Score*	If summary functional ability score is greater than 4, score 2.50.	____
Weight Loss	If lost 5 or more pounds in last 30 days *or* 10 or more pounds in last 180 days, score 2.26.	____
Shortness of Breath	If has shortness of breath, score 2.08.	____
Swallowing Problems	If has swallowing problems, score 1.81.	____
Male Sex	If male, score 1.76.	____
Body Mass Index	If BMI is less than 22 kg/m^2, score 1.75.	____
Congestive Heart Failure	If has CHF, score 1.57.	____
Age > 88 years	If age greater than 88, score 1.48.	____
	Total Score:	____

*To derive functional ability score, use MDS data for the following 7 items: bed mobility, transferring, eating, toileting, hygiene, locomotion on unit, and dressing. Each item is scored on a scale of 0 (no impairment) to 4 (high impairment), for a summary scale score ranging from 0–28.

If total score is:	Probability of dying within 1 year is approximately:
0–2	7%
3–6	19%
7–10	50%
11+	86%

---

[1]Derived from: Flacker, J. M., & Kiely, D. K. (1998). A practical approach to identifying mortality-related factors in established long-term care residents. *Journal of the American Geriatrics Society, 46,* 1012–1015.

National Hospice and Palliative Care Organization

General Medical Guidelines for Determining
Prognosis in Selected Non-Cancer Diseases

(adapted from National Hospice Organization, 1996,
updated to reflect common current practices)

The patient should meet all of the following criteria:

I.   The patient's condition is life limiting, and the patient and/or
     family know this
II. The patient and/or family have elected treatment goals directed
     toward relief of symptoms, rather than the underlying disease
III. The patient has either of the following:
     A. Documented clinical progression of the disease, which may
        include:
        1. Progression of the primary disease process as listed in
           the disease-specific criteria, as documented by serial phy-
           sician assessment, laboratory, radiologic, or other studies
        2. Multiple emergency department visits or inpatient hospi-
           talizations over the prior 6 months
        3. For homebound patients receiving home health services,
           nursing assessment may document decline
        4. For patients who do not qualify under 1, 2, or 3, a recent
           decline in functional status should be documented; clini-
           cal judgment is required
     B. Documented recent impaired nutritional status related to
        the terminal process:
        1. Unintentional, progressive weight loss of >10% over the
           prior 6 months
        2. Serum albumin <25 g/L may be a helpful prognostic
           indicator, but should not be used in isolation from other
           factors above

Highlights of Guidelines for Specific Diseases

Heart Disease:

I.   Intractable or frequently recurrent symptomatic heart failure, or
     intractable angina pectoris with heart failure
II. Patients should already be optimally treated with diuretics and
     vasodilators
III. Other factors contributing to a poor prognosis: symptomatic

arrhythmias, history of cardiac arrest and resuscitation or syncope, cardiogenic brain embolism, or concomitant human immunodeficiency virus disease

Pulmonary disease:

I. Severe chronic lung disease, documented by dyspnea at rest, fatigue, decreased functional ability, or increased exacerbation
II. Cor pulmonale or right heart failure
III. Hypoxemia at rest on supplemental oxygen
IV. Hypercapnia (pCO_2 >50 mm Hg)
V. Other factors contributing to a poor prognosis: unintentional continuing weight loss of >10% body weight over the preceding 6 months; resting tachycardia greater than 100/min

Dementia:

I. Severe dementia: unable to ambulate without assistance and unable to communicate meaningfully
II. Presence of medical complications: aspiration pneumonia, sepsis, intractable decubitus ulcers
III. Other factors contributing to a poor prognosis: unable to dress without assistance, unable to bathe properly, urinary and fecal incontinence

Human Immunodeficiency Virus disease:

I. $CD4^+$ count <25 cells/μL
II. Viral load >100 000 copies/mL
III. Life-threatening concomitant conditions
IV. Other factors contributing to a poor prognosis: chronic persistent diarrhea for 1 year; persistent serum albumin <25 g/L; concomitant substance abuse; age >50 years; decisions to forgo human immunodeficiency virus disease treatment; and symptomatic heart failure

Liver disease, advanced cirrhosis:

I. Both serum albumin <25 g/L, and either international normalized ratio >1.5 on no anticoagulants, or prothrombin time prolonged >5 seconds over control
II. At least 1 of the following: intractable ascites or hepatic encephalopathy, spontaneous bacterial peritonitis, hepatorenal syndrome, recurrent variceal bleeding
III. Other factors contributing to a poor prognosis: progressive malnutrition, muscle wasting, continued active alcoholism, hepatocellular carcinoma, and hepatitis B surface antigen positivity

Renal disease:

   I.   Creatinine clearance <0.17 mL/s (10 mL/min) and serum creatinine greater than 707.2 μmol/L (8.0 mg/dL)

   II. End stage renal disease discontinuing dialysis, or dialysis-eligible but refusing, and therefore with uremia, oliguria, intractable hyperkalemia, uremic pericarditis, hepatorenal syndrome, and/or intractable fluid overload

   III. Other factors contributing to a poor prognosis: mechanical ventilation, malignancy of other organ systems, chronic lung disease, advanced cardiac disease, advanced liver disease, sepsis, immunosuppression/acquired immunodeficiency syndrome, albumin <35 g/L, cachexia, platelet count <25 x 10^9/L, age >75 years, disseminated intravascular coagulation, gastrointestinal bleeding

Acute stroke and coma:

   I.   Coma or persistent vegetative state, beyond 3 days' duration, or

   II. In postanoxic state, coma or severe obtundation, accompanied by severe myoclonus, persisting beyond 3 days past the anoxic event, or

   III. Comatose patients with any 4 of the following on day 3 of coma (97% mortality by 3 months): abnormal brain stem response, absent verbal response, absent withdrawal response to pain, serum creatinine >132.6 μmol/L (1.5 mg/dL), age >70 years, or

   IV. Dysphagia severe enough to prevent the patient from receiving foods and fluids necessary to sustain life (patient not using artificial nutrition/hydration)

Chronic, after stroke:

   I.   Poor functional status, as evidenced by Karnofsky score of <50%, with evidence of recent decline

   II. Medical complications related to debility and progressive clinical decline, such as: aspiration pneumonia, upper urinary tract infection, sepsis, refractory stage 3-4 decubitus ulcers, or fever recurrent after antibiotics

   III. Also weigh: post-stroke severe dementia; age >70 years; poor nutritional status

Adapted with permission from: National Hospice Organization. *Medical Guidelines for Determining Prognosis in Selected Non-Cancer Diseases;* 1996.

(Reprinted) JAMA, February 21, 2001—Vol 285, No. 7 929

Appendix B

Approaches to Pain Assessment and Treatment

┌───┐
│ Resident _____ Date _____ Time _____   │
└───┘

Verbal Pain Scale

Ask the resident: "On a scale of 0 to 10, with 0 being no pain, 1–3 being mild pain, 4–6 being moderate pain, and 7–10 being severe pain, with 10 being the worst pain you can imagine, what number would you say best describes your pain right now?"

0:	No Pain
1–3:	Mild Pain
4–6:	Moderate Pain
7–10:	Severe Pain

┌───┐
│ Resident _____ Date _____ Time _____   │
└───┘

Verbal Pain Scale

Ask the resident: "On a scale of 0 to 5, with 0 being no pain, 1 being mild pain, 2 being discomforting pain, 3 being distressing pain, 4 being horrible pain, and 5 being excruciating pain, what number would you say best describes your pain right now?"

0 — No Pain
1 — Mild
2 — Discomforting
3 — Distressing
4 — Horrible
5 — Excruciating

Resident _____ Date _____ Time _____

Visual Pain Scale

Say to the resident: "The line below represents "no pain" at one end and "worst possible pain" at the other end. Point to or draw a mark on the point on the line that best describes your pain right now."

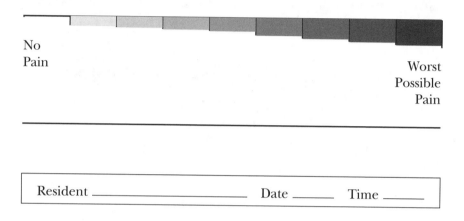

No
Pain

Worst
Possible
Pain

Resident _____ Date _____ Time _____

Visual Pain Scale

Say to the resident: "The line below runs from 0 to 10, with 0 meaning "no pain" and 10 meaning the "worst possible pain." Point to or draw a mark in the box that best describes your pain right now."

0	1	2	3	4	5	6	7	8	9	10
❑	❑	❑	❑	❑	❑	❑	❑	❑	❑	❑

No
pain

Worst
possible
pain

Resident _____ Date _____ Time _____

Visual Pain Scale*

Say to the resident: "There are six faces below. The first face is a smiling, happy face, representing no pain. The last face is a sad, crying face, representing severe pain. The four middle faces are somewhere in between. Point to or draw a mark beside the face that best describes your pain right now."

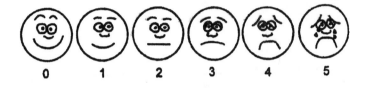

  0   1   2   3   4   5

*The Wong-Baker Faces Pain Rating Scale

| Resident _____ | Date _____ | Time _____ |

Observed Discomfort Scale*

For use with residents who are unable to communicate verbally. Keep copies of this form in the resident's chart and complete on a regular basis, using your observations of the resident's demeanor, expressions, movements, etc. Scores can range from 0 (no discomfort observed) to 27 (extreme discomfort observed). A 5-minute observation period should be adequate to identify discomfort while ruling out transitory and meaningless gestures and postures. The form can be used to assess the efficacy of comfort-promoting practices.

	None	Minimal	Moderate	Extreme
NOISY BREATHING (difficult, strenuous, loud, gasping)	0	1	2	3
NEGATIVE VOCALIZATIONS (including disapproving, unpleasant, muttering, or repetitious words of sounds)	0	1	2	3
CONTENT, PLEASANT, OR PEACEFUL EXPRESSION (relaxed, positive, no tension around mouth, at ease, serene)	3	2	1	0
SAD FACIAL EXPRESSION (troubled, hopeless, sunken hang-dog look, lips trembling, downward gaze)	0	1	2	3
FRIGHTENED FACIAL EXPRESSION (alarmed, pleading, eyes wide open, mouth open, forehead wrinkles)	0	1	2	3
FROWNING, STRAINED, STERN, OR DISPLEASED FACIAL EXPRESSION (scowling; angry; lips pressed together; hard, penetrating stare)	0	1	2	3
RELAXED BODY LANGUAGE (casual, leisurely, restful, idle, taking things in)	3	2	1	0
TENSE OR RIGID BODY (gripping something/someone, strained, inflexible, knees pulled up)	0	1	2	3
FIDGETING MOVEMENTS (restless, impatient, squirming, jittery, tugging at or rubbing body parts)	0	1	2	3

SCORE: _____

*Derived from: Hurley, A. C., Volicer, B. J., et al. (1992). Assessment of discomfort in advanced alzheimer patients. *Research in Nursing and Health, 15,* 369–377.

Resident _____ Date _____

Pain Assessment Form

(to be completed initially and quarterly)

Pain Medication: ❏ Routine   ❏ PRN   ❏ None

Medication/Dose/Interval: _____

_____

_____

Diagnosis: _____

Allergies: _____

Circle best responses:

Alert and Oriented?	Verbalizes Pain?	Present Pain Intensity
0 = no	Y = yes	0 = no pain
1 = ×1	N = no	1 = mild pain
2 = ×2		2 = discomforting pain
3 = ×3		3 = distressing pain
		4 = horrible pain
		5 = excruciating pain

Nursing Observations (circle all that apply):

A = complaining	H = restiveness	O = tense fingers
B = crying	I = wrinkled brow	P = withdrawal
C = moaning	J = facial grimacing	Q = sleep
D = fidgeting	K = sad/worried look	R = insomnia
E = restless	L = frightened appearance	S = anger
F = muscle rigidity	M = wincing	T = depression
G = agitation	N = guarding	

Pain Site/Location

A = upper back pain
B = lower back pain
C = chest pain
D = headache pain
E = hip pain

F = incision pain
G = joint pain _____
H = upper abdominal pain
I = lower abdominal pain
J = other _____

Description of Pain:

A = achy
B = dull
C = sharp
D = upon movement
E = upon touch

F = stabbing
G = throbbing
H = radiating
I = burning
J = itching

Frequency of Pain:

A = daily

B = less than daily

Time of Pain:

A = morning
B = afternoon
C = dinnertime
D = evening

E = bedtime
F = all times
G = intermittent
H = night

What causes or increases pain?

_____

_____

_____

_____

PAIN ASSESSMENT AND TREATMENT FORM

Name: _____   Room #: _____   MR #: _____

Section I: Current Status

1. Are there any diagnosis or treatments that predispose the
    resident to pain? ❏ Yes   ❏ No

    If yes, list: _____

    _____

2. Where is the resident's pain? _____

    _____

3. Ask the resident to describe his/her pain (e.g., aching, sharp,
    occasional, continuous, tender, numb): _____

    _____

4. If unable to self report, document behaviors indicative of pain
    (e.g., crying, groaning, grimacing): _____

    _____

5. Is the resident currently taking medication to treat pain? _____

    _____

    If yes, are these causing any adverse reactions? _____

    _____

Section II: Pain History

1. What makes the resident's pain better? (e.g., exercise,
    repositioning, hot packs, medications): _____

    _____

    _____

2. What makes the resident's pain worse? _____

_____

_____

3. Timing of the resident's pain (e.g., onset, duration, frequency,
    constant or intermittent) _____

_____

4. What time of day is the pain worse?

    ❒ Morning   ❒ Afternoon   ❒ Evening   ❒ Night

    Does this vary? If so, explain: _____

_____

5. How does the pain interfere with the resident's daily activities? __

_____

6. What pain medications has the resident taken in the past, and
    how did these work? _____

_____

Section III: Pain Scale

1. Use the following pain scale to assess the resident's pain. Circle
    the appropriate level.

No Pain	Mild	Moderate	Distressing	Horrible	Unbearable
0	2	4	6	8	10

Is this assessment from the resident's self-report? ❒ Yes   ❒ No

If no, is it from:

❒ licensed nurse assessment ❒ family assessment ❒ other _____

Section IV: Nursing Procedure

1. If the pain is mild (i.e., 2 or less), and the resident is not already taking a pain medication, try PRN standing order (check for contraindications or allergies prior to implementing standing orders).

2. If the pain is moderate or greater, or if mild pain was not relieved by PRN medication, contact the physician, physician assistant, or nurse practitioner for the suggested medication treatment protocol.

Name of MD/PA/NP contacted: _____

Date contacted: _____

Nurse contacting prescriber: _____

Response or order: _____

_____

Other comments: _____

_____

_____

Completed by: _____ Date: _____

Nurse's/Team Leader's Palliative/ Comfort Care Planning Worksheet

(for residents with a terminal prognosis, severe pain, or other distressing symptoms)

Resident Name: _____ Room: _____ Date: _____

Check each sign present:

❐ Dependent in all ADLs	❐ Increased use of PRN meds	Additional signs w/ advanced dementia:
❐ Swallowing problems	❐ Increased pain	❐ Uses only a few words
❐ Weight loss >10% TBW	❐ Stopped eating/ drinking	❐ Doesn't walk, sit, stand, smile
❐ Increased shortness of breath	❐ Talking about death more	❐ Trouble swallowing
❐ CHF	❐ Withdrawn	❐ Recurrent pneumonia

❐ Other severe symptoms (list): _____ ❐ Recent hip fracture
❐ Meets National Hospice Organization criteria for: _____

Has this resident been evaluated for causes of the above changes?

Circle one: YES   NO

Medically, is this resident appropriate for a palliative care plan?

Circle one: YES   NO

Special needs / personalized approaches that might be helpful for
PAIN: _____

_____

_____

Special needs / personalized approaches for OTHER SYMPTOMS: __

_____

_____

Special needs / personalized approaches for EMOTIONAL/
SPIRITUAL NEEDS:

_____

_____

_____

Special needs / personalized approaches for FOOD, DRINK, AND
PERSONAL CARE: _____

_____

_____

Special needs/personalized approaches for MOUTH CARE: _____

_____

Special needs/personalized approaches for BOWEL REGIMEN: _____

_____

Other comments: _____

_____

_____

_____

Nursing Representative: _____ Date: _____

SOCIAL WORKER'S PALLIATIVE/ COMFORT CARE PLANNING WORKSHEET

Resident Name: _____ Room: _____ Date: _____

Obtained resident's/family's verbal permission for goal of palliative or comfort care? _____

Communication about end-of-life concerns: _____

_____

_____

_____

_____

_____

_____

List all participants in the decision-making process and their relationship to the resident: _____

_____

_____

_____

_____

_____

Advance Directives and Orders:

	Done	Under Discussion	Discussed/ Declined
DNR order:	❏	❏	❏
Do Not Hospitalize Order	❏	❏	❏
Living Will:	❏	❏	❏
HCPOA	❏	❏	❏
Hospice referral:	❏	❏	❏

Other: _____

Social Worker: _____ Date: _____

Orders to Consider for a Comfort Care Plan

Comfort Care Plans are designed to meet the needs of residents who are approaching death, and plans are implemented after a medical provider has determined that the resident has an incurable, life-limiting condition and the resident and/or their family decision maker have agreed that treatment should focus on comfort and quality of life. Referral to hospice for collaborative care is recommended.

Overall Comfort:

- Do Not Attempt Resuscitation

- Do Not Hospitalize unless resident's comfort cannot be achieved

- Discontinue the following medications:

Pain Management: Short-Acting Treatment:

- nonpharmacologic pain management options—positioning, warm packs, cold packs, massage, listening, counseling, distraction

- morphine elixir 5–20 mg PO or SL q 1–4 hours

- hydromorphone 2 mg PO q 1–4 hours

- oxycodone 5–10 mg PO q 1–4 hours

Pain Management: Long-Acting Treatment:
Start with the lowest dose for residents who have never taken opioids before. (Dosage of all long-acting opioids should be calculated based on 24-hour usage of short-acting opioids)

- rocecoxib 25 mg PO qd (non-opioid)

- acetominophen 1000 mg PO q 8 hours (non-opioid)

- fentanyl patch 25 mcg to skin every 72 hours (onset of effect 24–48 hours)

- MS Contin; start with 15 mg q 12 hours

- OxyContin; start with 10 mg q 12 hours

- Methadone; may begin scheduled dosing at 5 mg TID

SHORTNESS OF BREATH:

- oxygen

- upright positioning

- morphine elixir 5–20 mg PO or SL q 2–4 hours PRN shortness of breath with anxiety

- lorazepam 1–2 mg PO or dissolved in 2 cc water sublingual q 2 hours PRN shortness of breath

- scopalamine 1.5 mg transdermal patch q 72 hours for thick secretions

NAUSEA:

- promethazine 12.5–25 mg PO or PR q 4 hours

- metaclopromide 10 mg PO q 4 hours

- lorazepam 1–2 mg PO or dissolved in 2 cc water sublingual q 2 hours PRN nausea

- haloperidol 0.5–2 mg PO q 4 hours PRN nausea

ANXIETY:

- lorazepam 0.5–2 mg PO, or dissolved in 2 cc water submucosal q 2 hours PRN for anxiety; NOT TO BE USED FOR DELIRIUM, unless cause of delirium has been investigated and major tranquilizer is in place first. Then a benzodiazepine may be used in small amounts temporarily for acute agitation.

DELIRIUM:

- haloperidol 0.5–2.0 mg PO q 6 hours

- risperidone 0.5–2.0 mg PO q 6 hours

- quetiapine 25–50 mg PO q 12 hours

EMOTIONAL AND SPIRITUAL NEEDS:

- Arrange for resident to be in a single room, quiet, with resident's familiar objects and belongings, and comfortable furniture for family members

- Unlimited visiting hours

- Request favorite music in room
- Request clergy or special friends to visit

FOOD, DRINK, AND PERSONAL CARE:

- Offer resident favorite beverages or foods as tolerated
- Turn or reposition every 2 hours for comfort; assess whether repositioning *causes* discomfort and modify order appropriately
- Bed bath/personal care as needed to ensure cleanliness

MOUTH CARE:

- Mouth care with water swab or mint/peroxide swab at least every 2 hours

BOWEL REGIMEN:

- Sennakot S (senna and doccusate sodium) 1–2 tablets PO qd; increase to BID and go up to 8 tablets per 24 hours if needed
- bisacodyl 10 mg PO or PR qd
- sorbitol 15–60 cc PO qd; if high impaction, titrate up to q 4 hours or until resident has BM

FAX or Phone Call
Cover Sheet

Date
_____

Number of pages
including cover sheet
_____

TO: **FROM:**

Phone   **Phone**
Fax Phone   **Fax Phone**
_____   _____

REMARKS: ❐ Urgent   ❐ Reply ASAP   ❐ Please Comment

Pain Assessment for: (Name)_____
(DOB) __/__/__   (MR#) _____

Diagnoses:

Pain severity:

Pain description:

Impact on function:

CURRENT TREATMENT (include dose, PRN doses given in past 48 hours):

RECOMMENDATIONS:

1.

2.

3.

RN Signature: _____

Pharmacist Signature: _____

MD RESPONSE:

_____

_____

_____

MD Signature: _____ **Print Name:**_____

Date: _____   **DEA #:** _____

NURSE WORKSHEET FOR PHONE CALL INTERVENTIONS

Before calling the prescriber, have the resident's chart and all the following information on hand. Be brief and specific in your report, but be prepared to supply additional information if it is needed. Ask the prescriber if you may call back if the new order does not give adequate pain relief.

Pain Assessment for (Name): _____

(DOB): __/__/__ (MR#): _____

Vital Signs: BP: ____ Pulse: ____ Temp: ____ Wt: ____

Pain Location/s: _____

Description (Quality): _____

Severity (0–10, 0–5, etc): _____

Diagnoses/Problem List: _____

Drug, dosage, and # of doses received of all analgesic medications in the past 24 hours: _____

Nonpharmalogical (complementary) interventions tried: _____

Allergies: _____

Suggestions for changes in management:

New meds/dosages/intervals: _____

Discontinue: _____

Nonpharmacologic (complementary) interventions: _____

Verbal Orders: _____

Nurse: _____ Date: _____ Time: _____

Prescriber: _____ Date: _____ Time: _____

IF RESIDENTS CANNOT COMMUNICATE THEIR PAIN VERBALLY, LOOK FOR NON-VERBAL CUES, SUCH AS CHANGES IN:

- Facial expressions
- Hand gestures
- Vocal expressions
- Breathing patterns
- Activity level
- Vital signs
- Body movements
- Self-care activities

POSSIBLE COMPLEMENTARY (NON-DRUG) TREATMENTS TO HELP RESIDENTS IN PAIN

- Prayer
- Reading
- Relaxation
- Music
- Exercise
- 1:1 Visits
- Immobilization
- TENS
- Deep breathing
- Special or "comfort" foods
- Recreation therapy
- Repositioning
- Diversion
- Massage
- Art
- Reminiscing
- Aromatherapy
- Elevation
- Diary/Journaling
- Animal therapy
- Quiet atmosphere
- Help w/ personal cleanliness
- Hot/cold applications

Equianalgesic Table and Usual Starting Doses

Drug	Approximate Equianalgesic Dose		Usual Starting Dose for Moderate to Severe Pain	
	IV/SQ	Oral	IV/SQ	Oral
Opioids				
*Morphine, IR (MSIR, Roxanol)	10 mg q 4 hrs	30 mg q 4 hrs	2–10 mg q 4 hrs	2.5–10 mg q 4 hrs (if renal function is impaired, start with oxycodone)
Morphine, controlled release (MS Contin, Oramorph)	NA	90–120 mg q 12 hrs	NA	30–120 mg q 12 hrs (start only after 24 hr dose is established w/ short-acting morphine)
Hydromorphone (Dilaudid)	1.5 mg q 4 hrs	7.5 mg q 4 hrs	0.75–1.5 mg q 4 hrs	6 mg q 4 hrs.
Oxycodone (Oxyfast)	NA	30 mg q 4 hrs	NA	10 mg q 4 hrs
Oxycodone, controlled release (OxyContin)	NA	60–90 mg q 12 hrs	NA	10 mg q 12 hrs (start only after 24 hr dose is established w/ short-acting oxycodone)
Methadone (Dolophine)	NA	3–5 mg q 6–8 hrs	NA	2.5–5 mg q 8 hrs
★Fentanyl Patch (Duragesic)	Microgram/hr dose of transdermal fentanyl $\approx$ 1/2 of mg/day dose of oral morphine up to 200 mg/day. Dosing q 72 hrs. Consult on conversions.		Not Recommended	25 mcg to skin every 72 hrs (do not start in an opioid-naive resident)
Meperidine (Demerol) *Not recommended—listed for conversion only*	100 mg q 3 hrs	300 mg q 2–3 hrs	*Not Recommended*	*Not Recommended*

Equianalgesic Table and Usual Starting Doses (*continued*)

Drug	Approximate Equianalgesic Dose		Usual Starting Dose for Moderate to Severe Pain	
	IV/SQ	Oral	IV/SQ	Oral
Combination Opioids				
Hydrocodone w/ acetaminophen (Vicodin, Lortab)	NA	Dose limited to a total of 4 gms acetaminophen in 24 hrs	NA	5–10 mg q 3–4 hrs
Oxycodone w/acetaminophen (Percocet, Tylox)	NA		NA	5–10 mg q 3–4 hrs
Codeine w/ acetaminophen	NA		NA	30–60 mg q 3–4 hrs

*May use for pain or shortness of breath.

★Transdermal fentanyl is useful for patients with stable pain who cannot take oral medications. When applied initially, maximum analgesia may not be obtained for up to 24 hours, therefore previous analgesic should be continued for 12 hours to ensure a smooth transition. Supplemental doses of a short-acting opioid should also be used as needed during the first 24 hours and subsequently to relieve breakthrough pain.

LONG-ACTING OPIOIDS: To calculate the dosage of a long-acting opioid, divide the total daily dose of opioids by 2, and give this dose BID, with a short-acting opioid for rescue.

Note: All doses must be individualized. Start with the lowest dose that seems prudent. Older patients generally experience a slightly greater peak effect and a longer duration of effect from opioid doses when compared with younger patients. Titrate dosage up with regular reassessments until clinically satisfactory pain control is achieved with minimal or acceptable side effects. Side effects may decrease after a few days or may require switching to another agent or using other medications to control the side effect.

Adjuvant Analgesics

Pain Source	Drug Class	Examples	Notes
Bone or Soft Tissue	*NSAIDs	Celecoxib (Celebrex)	100 to 200 mg PO BID; MAX 400 mg/day
		Rofecoxib (Vioxx)	12.5 to 50 mg PO QD; MAX 50 mg/day
		Ibuprofen (Advil, Motrin)	MAX 3200 mg/day
		Naproxen (Naprosyn)	500 mg q 12 hrs; Susp. 125 mg/5 cc
		Salsalate (Discalcid)	1000–1500 mg TID; MAX 4.5 gms/day
Visceral or Neuropathic	Corticosteroids	Dexamethasone (Decadron)	4 mg BID. Titrate to effective dose; MAX 16 mg/day. May cause GI upset
Nerve Damage or Dysaesthesia— continuous burning	Antidepressants	Desipramine (Norpramin)	10–100 mg divided or hs; start low & titrate up 10–20 mg/day every 4 days until effective or SE
		Nortriptyline (Pamelor)	10–100 mg divided or HS; Less sedating
Nerve Damage or Dysaesthesia— lancinating or "shooting" pain	Anticonvulsants	Gabapentin (Neurontin)	100 mg PO TID; increase every few days; MAX 3600+/day
		Carbamazepine (Tegretol)	200 mg PO BID; MAX 1200 mg/day. Sedating

*Limit the time prescribed to reduce the risk of GI bleeding.

Breakthrough Pain/Rescue Doses

GENERAL RULE FOR RESCUE OR BREAKTHROUGH DOSING: Use 10% of the 24-hour total dose of opioid every 3–4 hours.

DOSE ADJUSTMENT RULE FOR AROUND-THE-CLOCK DOSING IF RESCUE DOSE IS NOT CONTROLLING THE PAIN:

- If pain is 1–3 (on a scale of 0–10), dose escalation is no more than 25% of the current dose.

- If pain is 4–6 (on a scale of 0–10), dose escalation is 25–50% of current dose.

- If pain is 7–10 (on a scale of 0–10), dose escalation is 50–100% of current dose.

Bowel Management

- Every patient taking an opioid needs bowel medication—with adjustment up as opioid is titrated up—and daily monitoring.

- Encourage fluids, juice, and bran. May combine applesauce, prune juice, and raw fiber in "pudding" to taste and titrate as needed.

- Many patients will need a stool softener with gentle laxative, e.g., docusate 100 mg + casanthranol 30 mg (Pericolace) or senna concentrate 8.6 mg and docusate 50 mg (Senokot-S). Rx: 1–2 tablets PO QD-TID.

- If no bowel movement in any 24 hours period, add:

Milk of Magnesia	30–60 ml q hs
or Bisacodyl (Dulcolax)	10–15 mg PO q hs
or Sorbitol	15–60 ml QD-BID

- If not effective by 72 hours, perform rectal exam to check for impaction. If not impacted, try:

Bisacodyl suppository	10 mg
or Magnesium citrate	4–8 oz PO
or mineral oil	30–60 ml PO
or phosphate enema (Fleets) or warm water enema	

- If impacted, apply xylocaine ointment on rectum several minutes before disimpacting digitally. A laxative may be needed as well to complete the cleaning-out process.

Advance Care Planning Booklet for Nursing Home Residents

Advance Care Planning Booklet for Nursing Home Residents

WHAT IS ADVANCE CARE PLANNING?

CHOOSING THE BEST CARE FOR YOUR FINAL STAGE OF LIFE

What Is Important to Me in the Final Stage of My Life?

We want to offer you the very best care if you become seriously ill and are facing the final stage of your life. No one likes to think about death, but most people want to avoid suffering and to receive care that makes them feel comfortable and respected as their health declines. Many people also feel that they want to die a peaceful and natural death, in a quiet, familiar room, with friends and family around.

None of us knows what the future holds for us. Many people lose the ability to say what they want when they are dying. We recommend that *everyone* think about how they would like to be taken care of in the final stage of their life. This process is called "advance care planning." The nursing home staff, your physician, and those close to you need to know your ideas about the kind of care you want.

It may be helpful for you to think about and share the answers to these questions:

➢ If you are unable to make health care decisions for yourself, whom would you most like to make decisions for you?

➢ What are some of the things that make life worth living to you?

➢ If you found out you were going to die soon, what are the things you would want to take care of first?

➢ Do you have religious or spiritual ways to get ready for death? If so, what are they?

➢ Are there health problems you think are worse than death, such as living with severe pain, being totally physically dependent, or being unable to recognize or communicate with family or friends?

➢ If you knew you were dying, how would you want people to care for you?

If you want to write down answers to these questions, you can use the worksheet enclosed in this pamphlet.

Whether or not you write down your wishes, it is important to discuss your decisions with your doctors and nurses and with those close to you.

What Choices Do I Have?

You should think about the kind of care you would most want in the final stage of your life.

Some people would prefer care that helps them be as comfortable and peaceful as possible. They believe that "heroic" medical treatments (such as breathing machines or feeding tubes) interfere with a natural death.

Other people would like every possible heroic measure to be used to keep them alive as long as possible, even if it means more pain or discomfort.

"Heroic measures" will be used unless you say that you do not want them.

What Kind of Care Would You Want When You Are Dying?

Remember that it is important to make these decisions *now* and to share them with your health care team and your loved ones.

IF YOU WANT THE KINDS OF CARE DESCRIBED BELOW, IT IS ESPECIALLY IM-PORTANT THAT YOU LET YOUR HEALTH CARE PROVIDERS AND YOUR LOVED ONES KNOW

> ➤ COMFORT CARE: Doctors and nurses can do many things to keep you comfortable. Medicines can control pain and nausea. Oxygen can help with breathing problems. Nurses and aides can help by keeping your mouth moist, helping you change positions, or giving back rubs. You may also want to have visits from a minister, special music, favorite foods, or other special treats.

> ➤ HOSPICE CARE: Hospice is special care from nurses and others trained to work with dying patients and families. Hospice workers and volunteers focus on quality of life and specialize in helping dying individuals make the best use of whatever time they have remaining. In most cases, you can have hospice care in a nursing home.

YOU WILL RECEIVE THE KINDS OF CARE DESCRIBED BELOW UNLESS YOU LET YOUR HEALTH CARE TEAM KNOW THAT THIS IS NOT WHAT YOU WANT

> ➤ CPR AND BREATHING MACHINES: Cardiopulmonary resuscitation (CPR) will be attempted if you stop breathing or your heart stops.

Someone will press forcefully on your chest to make your heart pump and will blow air into your lungs.

Very few nursing home residents who get CPR can be brought back to life. In the rare chance you survive CPR, you will need to be moved to the hospital and placed on a breathing machine in the intensive care unit. This machine usually keeps people from talking and moving.

➤ FEEDING TUBE: If you stop eating, liquid feeding may be started by inserting a tube in your nose or stomach. You may not want tube feedings if you are dying or if you have end-stage Alzheimer's disease. Most dying patients lose their desire to eat and drink and are more comfortable without foods or liquids.

➤ HOSPITALIZATION: If you are dying, you may want to avoid going to the hospital, instead preferring to stay in your place of residence with familiar surroundings. Common illnesses like pneumonia can be treated in a nursing home. You may state that you don't want to go to the hospital or that you only want to go for treatments or comfort measures that cannot be provided in the nursing home.

How Can I Put My Wishes in Writing?

TELL YOUR DOCTOR OR NURSE ABOUT YOUR WISHES

➤ NAME A SURROGATE: This means that your doctor or nurse records in your chart the name of a person or persons you would like to help make health care decisions for you if you become unable to talk. *Doctors and nurses will talk with your family members unless you specify a certain family member you trust the most or someone else outside the family.*

COMPLETE LEGAL DOCUMENTS

➤ NAME A HEALTH CARE POWER OF ATTORNEY (HCPOA): A Health Care Power of Attorney gives your surrogate the legal power to make health care decisions for you if you cannot speak for yourself. A Health Care Power of Attorney is especially important for people who want someone other than a family member to make decisions. A HCPOA is *not* the same as Power of Attorney. The first is for making *health care* decisions, the second is for signing business documents.

➤ WRITE A LIVING WILL: This is a notarized and witnessed document specifying that if you become terminally ill or fall into a coma, you do not want extraordinary measures used to prolong your life. Your doctor or nurse can help explain the treatment options available to you.

Documents such as Living Wills or HCPOAs become effective only when you are incapable of making decisions for yourself. As long as you can understand and talk about your wishes, your doctors and nurses will ask you what you want.

ASK YOUR DOCTOR TO WRITE ORDERS IN YOUR CHART SPECIFYING YOUR WISHES. For example, you could:

➤ ASK FOR A DO-NOT-RESUSCITATE ORDER: This will prevent others from giving you CPR or placing you on a breathing machine.

➤ ASK FOR A COMFORT CARE OR HOSPICE CARE PLAN

May I Change My Mind About My Wishes?

Yes, you may always change your mind. Just tell your family and your doctor, and they will respect your new wishes. If you have written down your wishes, be sure to update your records by filling out a new form.

What Should I Do Now?

➤ Think about what care you want in the final stages of life.

➤ Share your ideas about your health care wishes with your family and your doctor and nurse.

➤ Tell your doctor or nurse the name of the person you would most trust to speak for you if you can't make your wishes known.

To help with this process, you may want to:

• Write down your thoughts, using the enclosed form.
• Ask the social worker to help you write a Living Will or appoint a Health Care Power of Attorney.
• Ask your doctor to write orders in your chart.

"My Thoughts on Advance Care Planning" Worksheet

You can use this worksheet to help you think about the kind of medical care you would want if you became too ill to communicate your wishes. You can also use it as a guide to help you gather your thoughts, so that you can talk to your family and your doctors and nurses.

1. *If you are unable to make health care decisions for yourself, whom would you most like to make decisions for you?*

    _____

2. *What are some of the things that make life worth living to you?*

    _____

    _____

    _____

    _____

    _____

3. *If you found out you were going to die soon, what are some of the personal things you would want to take care of (for example, people you would want to talk to or have visit)?* _____

    _____

    _____

    _____

4. *If you found out you were going to die soon, what are some of the practical matters that you would want to take care of (for example, business or legal issues, funeral planning)?* _____

    _____

    _____

5. *Do you have religious or spiritual ways to get ready for death? If so, what are they?* _____

_____

_____

_____

6. *Are there health problems that you think are worse than death, such as living with severe pain, with total physical dependency, or not being able to recognize or communicate with family and friends?* _____

_____

_____

_____

7. *If you knew you were dying, how would you want people to care for you besides medicine for comfort (for example, special music, prayers, readings, massage, etc)?* _____

_____

_____

_____

8. *If you were dying, which of the following approaches to treatment sounds most like what you would want? (You may choose more than one. If there are parts of the sentence that you don't agree with, you can cross those out.)*

❒ My main wish would be for care that will allow me to be comfortable, peaceful, and free from pain (including hospice care, if possible).

❒ I would want to go to the hospital for other treatments if necessary for comfort, but I would not want to be hooked up to life-support machines.

❒ If it were unclear whether a trial of life-support treatment would improve my chances of living, I would like to have a brief treatment period in the hospital, but would like the treatments stopped if there was no improvement.

☐ I would like all possible life-support treatments to prolong life as long as possible, even if those treatments made me uncomfortable.

☐ *If you prefer, use this space to put your own ideas into words:*

_____

_____

_____

9. *If you were dying and unable to eat, which of the following treatments do you think you would want?*

☐ I would **want** to have a tube inserted into my stomach, nose, or mouth to feed me.

☐ I would **not want** a feeding tube.

10. *Have you already filled out, or are you ready to fill out, a Living Will or a Health Care Power of Attorney?*

☐ Yes, Living Will

☐ Yes, Health Care Power of Attorney

☐ No

☐ Don't know right now, but would like to discuss it

11. *What are your fears, concerns, questions?* _____

_____

_____

Please note that this form is simply to help you think, plan, and discuss. *It is **not** a legal document*, although it maybe helpful to attach to your advance directive or put in your medical chart. ***Discuss these documents and give copies to your family and health care providers.***

Remember—no one can know your wishes unless you tell them!

Name ————————————————————————

Signature ——————————————————— Date ———

Health care provider discussing this with you ——————————

Health care provider's signature —————————————

Advance Care Planning Booklet for Families of Nursing Home Residents

Advance Care Planning Booklet for Families of Nursing Home Residents

WHAT IS ADVANCE CARE PLANNING?

HELPING FAMILIES CHOOSE THE BEST CARE FOR A LOVED ONE IN THE FINAL STAGE OF LIFE

What Is Important to Your Loved One in the Final Stage of Life?

We want to offer your loved one the very best care if she or he becomes seriously ill and is facing the final stage of life. No one likes to think about death, but most people want to avoid suffering and to receive care that makes them feel comfortable and respected as their health declines. Many people also feel that they want to die a peaceful and natural death, in a quiet, familiar room, with friends and family around.

None of us knows what the future holds for us. Many people lose the ability to say what they want when they are dying. We recommend that *everyone* think about how they would like to be taken care of in the final stage of their life. This process is called "advance care planning." The nursing home staff, your loved one's physician, and those close to your family member need to know your ideas about the kind of care your loved one wants. This booklet is designed to help you as you make health care decisions for your loved one if she or he is unable to participate in decision making or can only participate in a limited way.

It may be helpful for you to think about and share the answers to these questions:

➤ If your loved one is unable to make his own health care decisions, whom would he most like to make those decisions for him?

➤ What are some of the things that make life worth living for your loved one?

➤ If your loved one were going to die soon, what are the things that she would want to take care of first?

➤ Do you and/or your loved one have religious or spiritual ways to get ready for death? If so, what are they?

➤ Are there health problems that your loved one would think are worse than death, such as living with severe pain, being totally physically dependent, or being unable to recognize or communicate with family or friends?

➤ If your loved one were dying, how would you want people to care
for him?

If you want to write down answers to these questions, you can use the
worksheet enclosed in this pamphlet.

*Whether or not you write down your wishes, it is important to discuss your
thoughts with your family and your loved one's doctors and nurses. Telling
the doctors and nurses these things will ensure the best and most respectful
care for your loved one.*

What Choices Does My Loved One Have?

You should think about the kind of care your loved one would most
want in the final stages of life.
Some people would prefer care that helps them be as comfortable
and peaceful as possible. They believe that "heroic" medical treatments
(such as breathing machines or feeding tubes) interfere with a natural death.
Other people would like every possible heroic measure to be used
to keep them alive as long as possible, even if it means more pain
or discomfort.

*"Heroic measures" will be used unless you say that your loved one does not
want them.*

What Kind of Care Would Your Loved One Want When She or He Is Dying?

Remember that it is important to make these decisions *now* and to share
them with your family and your loved one's health care team.

IF YOUR LOVED ONE WOULD WANT THE KINDS OF CARE DESCRIBED BELOW, IT
IS ESPECIALLY IMPORTANT THAT YOU LET HEALTH CARE PROVIDERS AND FAMILY
MEMBERS KNOW

➤ COMFORT CARE: Doctors and nurses can do many things to keep
your loved one comfortable. Medicines can control pain and
nausea. Oxygen can help with breathing problems. Nurses and
aides can help by keeping the mouth moist, helping your loved
one change positions, or giving back rubs. Your loved one may
also want to have visits from a minister, special music, favorite
foods, or other special treats.

➤ HOSPICE CARE: Hospice is special care from nurses and others trained to work with dying patients and families. Hospice workers and volunteers focus on quality of life and specialize in helping dying individuals make the best use of whatever time they have remaining. In most cases, your loved one can have hospice care in a nursing home.

YOUR LOVED ONE WILL RECEIVE THE KINDS OF CARE DESCRIBED BELOW UNLESS YOU LET THE HEALTH CARE TEAM KNOW THAT THIS IS NOT WHAT YOU WANT:

➤ CPR AND BREATHING MACHINES: Cardiopulmonary resuscitation (CPR) will be attempted if your loved one stops breathing or her heart stops. Someone will press forcefully on her chest to make her heart pump and will blow air into her lungs.

Very few nursing home residents who get CPR can be brought back to life. In the rare chance your loved one survives CPR, she will need to be moved to the hospital and placed on a breathing machine in the intensive care unit. This machine usually keeps people from talking and moving.

➤ FEEDING TUBE: If your loved one stops eating, liquid feeding may be started by inserting a tube in his nose or stomach. Your loved one may not want tube feedings if he were dying or if he has end-stage Alzheimer's disease. Most dying patients lose their desire to eat and drink and are more comfortable without foods or liquids.

➤ HOSPITALIZATION: If your loved one is dying, she may want to avoid going to the hospital, instead preferring to stay in her place of residence with familiar surroundings. Common illnesses like pneumonia can be treated in a nursing home. You may state that your loved one does not want to go to the hospital or that she only wants to go for treatments or comfort measures that cannot be provided in the nursing home.

How Can You Put Your Loved One's Wishes in Writing?

TELL THE DOCTOR OR NURSE ABOUT YOUR LOVED ONE'S WISHES

➤ NAMING A SURROGATE: Whom do you believe your loved one would most trust to make health care decisions for him if he were unable to speak for himself? Give this person's name and contact information to your loved one's doctor or other primary care provider.

Talk With Your Loved One About Completing Legal Documents

> ➤ Naming a Health Care Power of Attorney (HCPOA): A Health Care Power of Attorney gives a surrogate the legal power to make health care decisions for your loved one if she cannot speak for herself. A Health Care Power of Attorney is especially important for people who want someone other than a family member to make decisions. A HCPOA is *not* the same as Power of Attorney. The first is for making *health care* decisions, the second is for signing business documents.

> ➤ Writing a Living Will: This is a notarized, witnessed document your loved one prepares that specifies that she does not want extraordinary measures used to prolong her life if she is dying. Your loved one's doctor or nurse can help explain the treatment options available to you and your family.

Documents such as Living Wills or HCPOAs become effective only when your loved one is incapable of making his own decisions.

As long as your loved one can understand and talk about his wishes, doctors and nurses will ask him what he wants.

Talk With Your Loved One and Her Doctor About Writing Orders in the Chart Specifying Your Loved One's Wishes. For example, You and your loved one could consider:

> ➤ Asking for a Do-Not-Resuscitate Order: This will prevent others from giving your loved one CPR or placing her on a breathing machine.

> ➤ Asking for a Comfort Care or a Hospice Care Plan

Can We Change Our Minds About Our Wishes?

Yes, you and your loved one can always change your minds. Just tell your family and your loved one's doctor, and they will respect your new wishes. If you or your loved one have written down your wishes, be sure to update medical records by filling out a new form.

What Should I Do Now?

> ➤ Think about what care you would want for your loved one in the

final stages of life, and talk with your loved one about her health care wishes if she is able to participate in a conversation.

➤ Share these ideas with your loved one's doctor or other primary care provider and nurse.

➤ Tell the doctor or nurse the name of the person your loved one would most trust to speak for him if he couldn't make his wishes known.

To help with this process, you may want to:

- Write down your thoughts, using the enclosed form.
- If possible, ask your loved one if she would like to write a Living Will or appoint a Health Care Power of Attorney.
- Talk with your loved one's doctor about writing orders in the chart.

"Advance Care Planning for My Loved One" Worksheet

You can use this worksheet to help think about the kind of medical care your loved one would want in the final stages of life. You can also use it as a planning guide to help you gather your thoughts, so that you can talk with your family and your loved one's doctors and nurses.

1. *If your loved one is unable to make her own health care decisions, who would she most like to make decisions for her?* _____

   _____

   _____

2. *What are some of the things that make life worth living for your loved one?* _____

   _____

   _____

   _____

   _____

3. *If your loved one were going to die soon, what are some of the personal things that would be important for him to take care of (for example, people he would want to talk with or have visit)?* _____

   _____

   _____

   _____

4. *If your loved one were going to die soon, what are some of the practical matters that she would want to take care of (for example, business or legal issues, funeral planning)?* _____

   _____

   _____

5. *Do you and/or your loved one have religious or spiritual ways to get ready for death? If so, what are they?* _____

_____

_____

_____

6. *Are there health problems that your loved one would think are worse than death, such as living with severe pain, with total physical dependency, or not being able to recognize or communicate with family and friends?* _____

_____

_____

_____

7. *If your loved one were dying, how would you want people to care for him (for example, special music, prayers, readings, massage, etc)?* _____

_____

_____

_____

8. *If your loved one were dying, which of the following approaches to treatment sounds most like what she would want? (You may choose more than one. If there are parts of the sentence that you don't agree with, you can cross those out.)*

❐ Her main wish would be for care in her place of residence that will allow her to be comfortable, peaceful, and free from pain (including hospice care, if possible).

❐ She would want to go to the hospital for other treatments if necessary for comfort, but would not want to be hooked up to life support machines.

❐ If it were unclear whether a trial of life-support treatment would improve his/her chances of living, she would like to have a brief treatment period in the hospital, but would like the treatments stopped if there was no improvement.

❐ She would like all possible life-support treatments to prolong life as long as possible, even if those treatments made her uncomfortable.

❐ *If you prefer, use this space to put your own ideas into words:* ___

_____

_____

9. *If your loved one were dying and unable to eat, which of the following treatments do you think he would want?*

❐ He would **want** to have a tube inserted into his stomach, nose, or mouth to feed him if he could not eat.

❐ He would **not want** a feeding tube if he could not eat.

10. *Has your loved one already filled out, or is ready to fill out, a Living Will or a Health Care Power of Attorney?*

❐ Yes, Living Will

❐ Yes, Health Care Power of Attorney

❐ No

❐ My loved one has not yet completed an advance directive but would like to discuss this option

11. *What are your fears, concerns, questions?* _____

_____

_____

Please note that this form is simply to help you think, plan, and discuss. *It is **not** a legal document*, although it would be helpful to attach this form to your loved one's advance directive or put in her medical chart. ***Discuss these documents, and give copies to your family and your loved one's doctor and nurse.***

Remember—no one can know your wishes or your loved one's wishes unless you tell them!

Name of loved one: _____ Date: ____

Names, signatures, and relationship to resident of persons discussing and completing this form: _____

_____

_____

Name and signature of health care professional discussing this document with you:

_____ Date: _____

Appendix E

Participants' Handouts

HANDOUTS FOR SESSION 1
ENVISIONING A GOOD DEATH

Homework

ENVISIONING A GOOD DEATH FOR ONE OF YOUR RESIDENTS

Pick one resident you believe is near the end of her life. As she nears death, are we paying attention to all of her needs?

☐ *Physical:* Is she getting the help she needs for pain, shortness of breath, mouth care, and personal cleanliness?

☐ *Emotional:* Have you tried to understand her concerns, fears, and wishes?

☐ *Social:* How can we support and nurture her connections with her family, friends, and staff who care about her? How can we support her family during this difficult time?

☐ *Spiritual:* What kind of religious or spiritual support does she want? Would she or her family like a visit from a minister? A prayer? A Bible reading? Special music?

➤ **What can you do right now to make these things happen for this resident?**

➤ **Tell another caregiver about what you did that helped.**

➤ **Try to get the resident's care plan changed to meet these needs.**

HANDOUTS FOR SESSION 2
RECOGNIZING THE FINAL PHASE OF LIFE

HOMEWORK

RECOGNIZING AND RESPONDING TO THE FINAL PHASE OF LIFE

Think about the residents you know, and:

☐ Identify at least one resident who is likely to die in the next few weeks or months. Think about ideal care for him during this time of preparation for dying.

- Have a conversation with other staff, family, or the resident that includes the words "dying," "die," or "death." For example, "Have you ever thought about how you would want your death to be when your time comes?"

- Do one thing to help the resident and family to make this time a special experience. For example, they may wish to have meals together, share memories, or have special religious ceremonies.

- Do one thing to provide emotional or spiritual support to this resident.

or

☐ Identify at least one resident who is actively dying or likely to die within days or weeks.

- Ask her about or observe what is making her uncomfortable. Remember that she may be having physical pain, but she also may be having difficulty with emotional and spiritual preparation for her death.

- Do one thing to make her more comfortable based on what you know about her.

➤ **What can you do right now to make these things happen for these residents?**

➤ **Tell another caregiver about what you did that helped.**

➤ **Try to get these residents' care plans changed to meet these needs.**

Recognizing the Final Phase of Life

Who needs a comfort care plan?

- Residents w/ life expectancy of less than 6 months
- Residents about whom you can say, "I wouldn't be surprised if she died within the next year."
- Residents with an incurable, progressive disease
- Anyone who wants a comfort care approach

Signs death might be near

- Needs more assistance with ADLs
- Weight loss
- Shortness of breath
- Swallowing problems
- Congestive heart failure
- Advanced Alzheimer's with hip fracture or pneumonia

Behaviors in the weeks to months before death

- Social withdrawal, less communication *or*
- Desire to address old conflicts
- Increased sleep; decreased intake of food and water
- Postponing death until a special event occurs
- Saying good-bye

Comforting residents who are actively dying

- Provide warm blankets or clothing
- Always assume resident's senses of hearing and touch are intact
- Take advantage of all opportunities to communicate and love
- Offer reassuring talk
- Give good mouth care
- Help with personal cleanliness (being careful not to cause pain)

Comforting residents who are actively dying (continued)

- Provide gentle massage
- Play music special to the resident
- Reassure and support family
- Treat for shortness of breath as needed
  - Give oxygen
  - Give low-dose morphine
  - Elevate head

HANDOUTS FOR SESSION 3
GRIEF AND LOSS: UNDERSTANDING AND SUPPORTING FAMILIES

HOMEWORK

GRIEF AND LOSS: UNDERSTANDING AND SUPPORTING FAMILIES

Think of the family members you know in the facility. Identify one family member who is struggling with preparation for the death of a loved one who is a resident here.

❒   Say to that family member, "I know this is a difficult time for you," and take time to listen and learn from his response.

❒   Tell the family member how special her loved one is to you, and tell her what you are doing to care for this resident.

❒   Ask him, "Is there anything more I can do to make this time easier for you or your loved one?"

❒   Do one thing that you sense will be comforting for that family member, for example offering a cup of coffee, helping arrange an overnight stay in the resident's room, or showing her how to touch her loved one in a way that is comforting.

➤   **What can you do right now to make these things happen for this family member?**

➤   **Tell another caregiver about what you did that helped.**

➤   **Try to get the resident's care plan changed to meet these needs.**

Grief and Loss:

Understanding and
Supporting Families

What do families want for their dying loved ones?

- Presence and support of staff
- Spiritual support
- Personal cleanliness/attention to details of their loved one's care
- Freedom from pain and discomfort
- Communication with staff

What can you offer grieving family members

- Be there
- Listen
- Offer your presence and concern

What are some family stresses during the dying process?

- Feelings of sadness, anger, or guilt
- Difficulty balancing a dying person's needs with other demands
- Changing of family roles
- Practical issues such as finances and funeral arrangements
- Old family conflicts that can surface during times of crisis
- Concerns about quality of care

What can you do to help grieving family members?

- Encourage the saying of good-byes
- Show family members how to touch or provide personal care for their loved ones
- Allow family members to give special, personalized care
- Listen to family members when they share their concerns or grief with you

What can you do to help grieving family members (continued)

- Recognize your own feelings
- Let family members know that you will provide the best care possible
- Attend funerals or other memorial services if possible
- Have memorial services at your facility; invite family members to attend

HANDOUTS FOR SESSION 4
ADVANCE CARE PLANNING

Note to Facilitator: In addition to the following materials, we suggest that you make copies of *Appendices C* and *D* available for session participants.

HOMEWORK

Advance Care Planning

Choose one resident who has *not* had any discussion of advance care planning. Do *one* thing to begin the advance care planning process, for example:

❐ ask the social worker, nurse, or physician to have this discussion if they have not yet done so, *or*

❐ talk with the resident about how she would like to be cared for if she were terminally ill; share this information and document in the chart, *or*

❐ set up a family meeting to discuss this issue, *or*

❐ clarify whether existing orders match your understanding of the resident's or the family's preferences, and ask for changes if needed

➤ **What can you do right now to make these things happen for this resident?**

➤ **Tell another caregiver about what you did that helped.**

➤ **Try to get the resident's care plan changed to meet these needs.**

Advance Care Planning

What is Advance Care Planning (ACP)?

- Process of planning one's final phase of life
- Should be done *before* a crisis occurs
- Includes thinking and discussing, looking at values and priorities
- Involves deciding what treatments one would want

ACP should result in a plan of care to:

- Make clear what treatments a resident wants or does not want (for example, CPR, hospitalization, tube feeding)
- Improve the resident's quality of life (for example, providing things the resident enjoys, offering comfort care, helping the resident to make the most of each and every day)

Who decides—resident or family?

- Try to include both resident and family
- Even residents with dementia can express preferences and participate with family in discussions
- A Health Care Power of Attorney or close family member can serve as a surrogate if residents cannot speak for themselves

What can you say?

- Ask resident about her values, priorities, and goals of care
- Let the individual know that you discuss this with all residents
- Reassure residents and families: let them know that you will respect their decisions and that you will always provide the best comfort care possible

Discussing end-of-life medical decisions

- CPR is an attempt to restart heart and breathing. Is usually unsuccessful. If resident survives, it offers no guarantee of recovering previous level of functioning.
- Ventilators (breathing machines) are used in an intensive care unit. A person will be sedated and unable to talk.

Discussing end-of-life medical decisions (continued)

- IV fluids and tube feedings provide nourishment when a person can no longer eat or drink.
  - Useful when resident will recover from current illness or when waiting for a special event
  - For a terminally ill resident, may prolong death and make resident less comfortable
  - Dying people generally want very little to eat or drink. This is not painful and they are not hungry or thirsty.

When is hospitalization appropriate?

- For evaluating treatable conditions when function can be restored (for example, a heart attack in a person who is not terminally ill)
- To give treatment only available in a hospital (for example, to pin a hip fracture)
- To give comfort care not available in the nursing home (for example, a nerve block for pain)

When is hospitalization *not* appropriate?

- When diagnosis and treatment can be done in the nursing home (for example, urinary tract infection)
- When the burden outweighs the benefit (for example, for a demented resident who would be frightened by a strange environment)
- When comfort care can be done in the nursing home

Social Workers/Admissions Officers and ACP

- Begin discussion on admission; ask about advance directives
- Ask about individual comfort care wishes
- Document conversations; communicate with other staff about residents' wishes
- Reassure that you will always give the very best care, regardless of treatment decisions

Certified Nursing Assistants and ACP

- You are often the first to hear about a resident's concerns or fears about death
- Reassure the resident you will help her or find others to help her
- Report comments about residents' fears or treatment wishes to the nurse

Nurses, NPs, PAs, MDs, and ACP

- Discuss with resident and families: diagnosis, prognosis, goals of care, individual preferences, and treatment options
- Record all discussions in the chart
- Reassure that you will always give the very best care possible
- Write medical orders (e.g., comfort care only, DNR, do not hospitalize)
- Refer to Hospice as appropriate

Talking With Residents & Families About Advance Care Planning—Things You Might Say:

"A federal law requires that we ask all new residents if they have a Living Will or a Health Care Power of Attorney. Do you have either one?"

"A doctor or nurse will discuss this more with you."

"We do not have to make all these decisions right now. We can talk about these issues again after you've had time to think about them and to talk with your family."

"Who would you trust to speak for you if you were ill and could not make decisions for yourself?"

"Are There Medical Treatments That You Fear or Do Not Want?"

"Help us to know what your mother would want if she could speak to us right now."

"Did your father have strong feelings about being on life support or heroic measures?"

"What Do You Hope Doctors and Nurses Can Do to Help You?"

"We discuss this with all residents because we want to honor their wishes."

"If your heart or breathing should stop, CPR can be attempted. Someone would do chest compressions and mouth-to-mouth resuscitation until emergency medical technicians arrive to place a breathing tube in your throat for assisted breathing. You will be taken to the hospital and attached to a ventilator. In most cases, CPR is not successful in reviving someone who is elderly or who is chronically or critically ill."

"We will always give you the very best care we can."

"What makes life worth living to you? What do you hope for now and in the future?"

"Where Do You Find Strength In Times Of Trouble?"

"Do you have religious or spiritual beliefs that help you make tough decisions?"

"Have you ever imagined what you would like your final days or hours to be like? Can you describe this?"

"We will always pay attention to your needs, and we promise to give you the best comfort care possible when you are dying."

HANDOUTS FOR SESSION 5
CHOICES ABOUT EATING AND DRINKING

HOMEWORK

HELPING RESIDENTS AND FAMILIES MAKE CHOICES ABOUT EATING AND DRINKING

Choose *one* resident who has a problem with intake—for example, a resident with weight loss, dehydration, poor oral hygiene, poor appetite, or swallowing difficulty:

❐ If you are a nurse:

- Assess treatable problems that might cause poor intake (e.g., depression, thyroid disease, medication effects, inadequate aide time to feed),

- Recommend one new intervention to improve eating and drinking if treatable problem is present, *or*

- Begin a discussion of treatment options if poor intake cannot be reversed. Listen for the family's or resident's ideas about the meaning of food from their emotional, cultural, or religious perspective.

❐ If you are a CNA:

- Observe the resident's intake, what foods the resident likes, and care needs during eating—think about why this resident is not eating much,

- Discuss your observations with a nurse,

- Plan one new approach to make eating or drinking more enjoyable, *or*

- Provide comfort to a resident who has naturally stopped eating or drinking.

➤ **What can you do right now to make these things happen for this resident?**

➤ **Tell another caregiver about what you did that helped.**

➤ **Try to get the resident's care plan changed to meet these needs.**

Choices About Eating and Drinking

Is stopping eating and drinking normal at the end of life?

- 2/3 of dying nursing home residents experience appetite loss
- Reduced need for nutritional intake is a natural part of the dying process
- Weight loss is to be expected in a dying resident
- Most dying residents are not hungry or thirsty

What happens when a resident drinks but doesn't eat?

- Can live for weeks to months
- Feelings of hunger are blunted
- Mental function may remain normal until just before death

What happens when a resident doesn't drink?

- Typically live 1–3 weeks
- Has a gradual loss of consciousness
- Death may be peaceful and comfortable
- Good mouth care is essential

What are reasons to recommend tube feeding or IV fluids?

- Can temporarily support a resident who has an acute illness but is not actively dying
- May improve comfort for residents who have hunger or thirst
- Can keep a resident alert temporarily while she awaits a special event
- Residents' or families' religious beliefs or feelings may require these treatments

What are reasons not to recommend tube feeding or IV fluids?

- Can lead to increased lung secretions, shortness of breath, edema, incontinence
- Lack of intake results in peaceful loss of consciousness
- May prolong the dying process
- Restraints may be used, causing distress for residents and families

GUIDELINES FOR EXCELLENT MOUTH CARE

PERFORM REGULARLY	May be required as often as every 1 to 2 hours for actively dying residents
REGULAR TOOTHBRUSHING FOR ALERT RESIDENTS	Use a small amount of toothpaste or mouthwash for residents who are more alert
MOUTHWASH	Offer alert residents alcohol-free mouthwash
FREQUENT "TREATS"	Offer alert residents hard candies, ice chips, sips of water, or water sprays; to prevent choking, give only when the resident is sitting up
REGULAR SWABS FOR LESS ALERT RESIDENTS	Use chlorhexidine 0.12% alcohol-free mouthwash or water on swabs at regular intervals for less alert residents
DENTURES	Remove and clean dentures regularly
MEDICATIONS	Reduce medications that cause dry mouth
THRUSH	Treat thrush with topical antifungals or a combination topical agent including an antifungal, viscous xylocaine, and diphenhydramine
CRUSTING	Use hydrogen peroxide diluted 1:1 with water; add a small amount of mint flavoring if possible
CRACKED LIPS	Treat dry, cracked lips with petroleum jelly, lip balm, or ointment with vitamins A&D

HANDOUTS FOR SESSION 6
PAIN MANAGEMENT

Note to Facilitator: In addition to the following items, we suggest that you make copies of materials in *Appendix B* available for all session participants.

HOMEWORK

PAIN MANAGEMENT: NURSES

Pick *one* resident who you fear is suffering from poorly treated pain.

☐ Ask about discomfort *and* observe pain behaviors to decide whether pain is present

☐ Choose a pain scale and ask the resident to rate the severity of pain

☐ Document your assessment and communicate to other team members

☐ Add "pain management" to the resident's care plan

☐ Plan treatment for the resident's pain

☐ Reassess pain severity using the same scale after treatment is begun

☐ Refine treatment plan until the resident reaches her goal of pain relief

➤ **What can you do right now to make these things happen for this resident?**

➤ **Tell another caregiver about what you did that helped.**

➤ **Try to get the resident's care plan changed to meet these needs.**

Remember: Routine assessment of *all* residents is important to find those who are in pain and to plan treatment.

HOMEWORK

Pain Management: CNAs and Other Nonlicensed Staff

Pick *one* resident who you fear is suffering from poorly treated pain.

- ☐ Ask about discomfort *and* observe pain behaviors to decide whether pain is present
- ☐ Use a pain scale to rate the severity of pain
- ☐ Report what you learn about pain or discomfort to the nurse
- ☐ Provide one comfort measure such as repositioning, soothing massage, or music
- ☐ Determine whether your comfort measure provides relief—if not, try a new approach, and if so, continue
- ☐ Recheck pain severity using the same scale after treatment is begun
- ☐ Report your successful treatment to the nurse and the CNA on the next shift.

- ➣ **What can you do right now to make these things happen for this resident?**
- ➣ **Tell another caregiver about what you did that helped.**
- ➣ **Try to get the resident's care plan changed to meet these needs.**

Remember: Routine assessment of *all* residents is important to find those who are in pain and to plan treatment.

Remember: CNAs are often the first staff members to notice when a resident is in pain! You are very important in helping to decrease pain and increase comfort for those you care for!

Pain Management

What are barriers to treating pain?

- Misconception that pain is inevitable, is part of the aging process, and cannot be managed
- Residents' unwillingness to "complain" about pain
- Fears about addiction
- **Most common barrier: Failure to ask about and assess pain**

How can you tell if a resident has pain?

- Ask every resident routinely!
- Use a pain scale if possible
- Observe the resident, looking for non-verbal clues
  - changes in behavior, vital signs
  - expressions of distress or withdrawal
- Review diagnoses—are any of them painful conditions?

How can you assess pain in residents with dementia?

- Ask them—4 out of 5 residents with dementia can report pain if asked
- Ask about pain "right now"
- Look for changes in
  - breathing
  - vocalizations
  - facial expressions
  - behaviors

Steps for successful pain management

- Regularly ask about/assess pain and discomfort
- Use a pain scale
- Review treatment history and current medications
- Use both medications and nondrug (complementary) treatments

Steps for successful pain management (continued)

- As a general rule, use scheduled meds instead of PRN meds
- Reassess pain after giving treatment
- Adjust treatment plan as needed
- Work as a team: CNAs, nurses, doctors, and other staff members each play an important role in successful pain management

Nurses and Pain Management

Different types of pain require different treatments

- Somatic—localized tissue discussion
  - e.g., arthritis, bone pain, pain after surgery, trauma
- Visceral—stretching internal organs
  - e.g., bowel obstruction, angina, urinary retention, constipation
- Neuropathic—injury to nerves
  - e.g., diabetic foot pain, shingles, pinched nerves

Important issues in medication use

- Scheduled dosing, not PRN
- Begin with short-acting dose. Once this works, switch to long-acting dose
- Use short-acting medications for breakthrough pain
- After giving medication, assess response

Important issues in medication use (continued)

- Increase dose and/or frequency until desired effect is achieved or until the resident experiences side effects
- Give dose before pain becomes severe
- Bowel regimen starts when opioids start

Talking with physicians

■ When you find that a resident is in pain, call her/his physician. Be prepared to give:
  ■ vital signs
  ■ severity (use pain scale if possible)
  ■ problem list and description of pain
  ■ medications already tried
  ■ your suggestions for treatment

Working with CNAs

■ Remember the vital role that CNAs play in pain management
  ■ They are at the bedside and often the first to notice signs of pain

■ Encourage CNAs to report signs of pain

■ Provide feedback to CNAs regarding changes in the treatment plan

■ Encourage CNAs to provide feedback about effects of treatment

CNAs and Pain Management

The importance of CNAs in pain management

- CNAs are at the bedside
- CNAs are often the people most likely to notice when a resident is acting differently or showing signs of pain
- CNAs' personal relationships with residents can be very helpful in pain management
- CNAs should take an active role in pain management

Examples of comfort measures CNAs can offer

- Supportive talk
- Gentle touch
- Music
- Soft lighting
- Decreased noise

Examples of comfort measures CNAs can offer (continued)

- Warm or cold packs, if OKed by nurse
- Massage
- Repositioning
- Soothing activities
- Prayer and spiritual support

Examples of comfort measures CNAs can offer (continued)

- Listening and conversation
- Favorite foods or drinks
- Help with personal cleanliness
- Reminiscing
- A walk

Helping residents with pain management

- Ask about both pain and discomfort
- Ask, "Where does it hurt?" "What makes it better?"
- Report what you observe to the nurse
- When you find something that works, let the CNA on the next shift know
- Work as a team with other staff members

HANDOUTS FOR SESSION 7
EMOTIONAL AND SPIRITUAL CARE

HOMEWORK

HELPING RESIDENTS WITH THEIR EMOTIONAL AND SPIRITUAL NEEDS

Choose *one* resident who is near the end of his life and is likely to have unmet emotional or spiritual needs. A resident with unmet needs may be someone who seems distressed, sad, or angry even when you try to help him.

❏ Start a conversation with this resident using phrases like these:

- "I know you are upset by something. Would you like to talk about it with me?"

- "It must be hard for you to be so sick, and not see yourself getting any better."

- "I know the doctor told you that you may not have long to live. Is there anything you want to do or anyone you wish to see?"

❏ Based on what you know about the resident, provide one change to meet an emotional or spiritual need. This might include:

- playing music that he prefers

- placing familiar objects with special meaning in her room

- inviting special visitors

- helping with a religious ceremony or ritual from the resident's own tradition

- offering a prayer or scripture reading

- sitting quietly or holding hands

- offering to organize a team of family and volunteers to sit with an actively dying resident who fears being alone

- offering to help him accomplish any last wishes

➤ **What can you do right now to make these things happen for this resident?**

➤ **Tell another caregiver about what you did that helped.**

➤ **Try to get the resident's care plan changed to meet these needs.**

Emotional and Spiritual Care

Helping residents with their spiritual and emotional needs

■ The ministry of presence is the most powerful comfort you can offer!

Some emotional concerns at the end of life

- How will I die?
- Will it be painful?
- Will I be taken care of?
- Will I be alone?
- What will happen to my family after I die?
- Are there things I want to do or say before I die?

Some spiritual concerns at the end of life

- Why am I dying?
- Where will I go after death?
- What has been meaningful about my life?
- How can I find meaning in my death?
- How can I be spiritually ready for my death?

How can you offer emotional support?

- Be with the resident and family
- Listen with full attention
- Be sympathetic
- Accept them, wherever they are, understanding that this is a difficult time for them

How can you offer emotional support? (continued)

- Help them enjoy life and make the most of each remaining day
- Allow them choices in routines and care
- Support special relationships the dying person has with staff, family, or friends

How can you offer spiritual support?

- Listen for spiritual language and concerns
- Don't offer "easy answers"
- Allow questions and anger without judgment
- Offer prayers, sacraments, religious music, etc., that are special to the resident

How can you offer spiritual support? (continued)

- Offer to contact the resident's preferred clergy member or a hospice chaplain
- Encourage the resident and family to reminisce
- Assure the resident that she or he will not be abandoned or forgotten, and that they will be missed

Issues to consider

■ Are you meeting the resident's physical needs?
  ■ Residents who are in pain, uncomfortable, or dirty will be less able to cope with their emotional and spiritual concerns
■ Does the resident want to talk about her approaching death?
■ What is the resident's cultural or religious background?

Issues to consider (continued)

■ What is the resident's emotional and spiritual state?
■ What are the resident's spiritual resources and inner strengths?
■ Who are the resident's social supports?

As you work with dying residents, remember

- Even people who cannot talk about spiritual concerns (for example, someone with advanced dementia) can respond to music, prayer, or touch
- Residents who are angry or in denial are defending themselves from emotional pain; try to respect and support them, wherever they may be

As you work with dying residents, remember

- Distinguish between your beliefs and the beliefs and needs of the resident
- Acknowledge—to residents, families, and yourself—the emotional and spiritual intensity of dying
- Excellent emotional and spiritual care creates good memories and promotes healing for family and staff

TALKING WITH RESIDENTS ABOUT EMOTIONAL AND SPIRITUAL CONCERNS—THINGS YOU MIGHT SAY:

"I know this is hard for you."

"I care about you and I'm here if you want to talk about anything."

"It must be hard to be so sick. Do you have any concerns about what is going to happen to you?"

"ARE YOU A RELIGIOUS OR SPIRITUAL PERSON?"

"Do you have any beliefs that help you through difficult times?"

"What has given your life meaning?"

"I know you are upset by something. Would you like to talk about it with me?"

"DO YOU HAVE ANY THOUGHTS ABOUT WHY THIS IS HAPPENING?"

"I understand that this is a very difficult time for you."

"I LOVE YOU."

"Would you like me to sit and pray with you?"

"How have you coped with hardship in your life?"

"I know the doctor told you that you might not have long to live. Is there anything you want to do or anyone you wish to see?"

"IF YOUR TIME TO DIE SHOULD COME SOON, DO YOU FEEL READY?"

"Have you ever experienced the death of a loved one? What was that like?"

"Who could I ask to come see you during this difficult time—special friends, clergy, family?"

"You are very special to me. I have enjoyed knowing you and caring for you."

"I will always remember you."

"I WILL MISS YOU."

A Caregiver's Prayer

May I offer my presence and care unconditionally, knowing that I may meet ingratitude, indifference, anger, and anguish. May I find the inner resources to truly be able to give. May I offer love, knowing that I cannot control the course of life, suffering, or death. May I view my own limits with compassion, just as I see the suffering of others.

HANDOUTS FOR SESSION 8
CARING FOR THE CAREGIVERS:
TAKING CARE OF YOURSELF EMOTIONALLY

HOMEWORK

CARING FOR THE CAREGIVERS:
TAKING CARE OF YOURSELF EMOTIONALLY

Read through the following choices. Pick *one* that would be the most challenging for you, and make one change to care for yourself or for someone who works with you.

❐ When trying to give good care to a suffering or dying resident, do you feel valued and supported by other people who work here?

- Think of one way a friend at work has helped you, and offer this same help to someone else in your facility

- Think of one way someone at work has supported you when a resident was dying, and thank them for it

❐ When trying to give good care to a suffering or dying resident, do you find strength from family, good friends, church, or other sources?

- Think of one thing you can do to reach out for strength for yourself the next time a resident is dying

❐ When a resident has died and you feel sad, do you have ideas about how to remember them with others?

- Talk with a staff member, a family member, or another resident about your sadness over the loss of the person who died

- Create a memory book for your facility

- Ask for time off to attend the funeral of a resident who you cared for

- Hold a meeting to discuss what would help staff when a resident dies

➤ **What can you do right now to make these things happen for *you*?**

➤ **Tell another caregiver about what you did that was helpful to *you*.**

➤ **Try to do something each day that helps meet *your* needs.**

Caring for the Caregiver

Taking Care of
Yourself Emotionally

Caring for dying residents can be very stressful

- People you care for die
- You see people who are sad, lonely, or in pain
- You have a heavy workload, with many residents to care for
- Family members of dying residents are also experiencing many difficult emotions that can affect you

Caring for dying residents can be very rewarding

- You help dying residents be clean, comfortable, and peaceful
- You work with and support other staff
- You help residents have a good death
- Your work helps you appreciate the value of life every day
- You share special moments with people you care for and love

How can you cope with working with people who are dying?

- Remember your own sources of strength
- Find support from others
- Feel proud of your commitment to this valuable work
- Look for continuing educational opportunities in end-of-life care

How can you give and get support from your coworkers?

- Ask for help when you find that caring for a dying resident or a family member is difficult
- Share your worries and grief with someone you trust
- Stop and offer support to a coworker who is having a difficult time
- When a resident is dying, ask what you can do to help another team member

How can you say good-bye?

- Let dying residents know that they are special to you and that you have enjoyed caring for them
- When a resident dies, let other residents and staff know
- Take time to tell stories and share feelings with your coworkers
- Participate in memorial services